Keto AF
Coloring Book

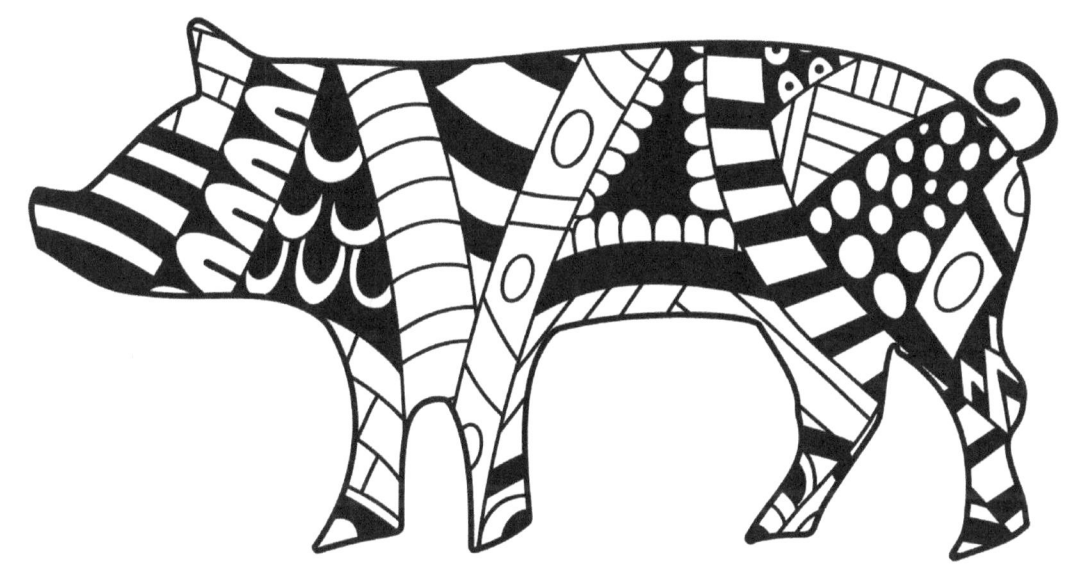

Cora Delmonico

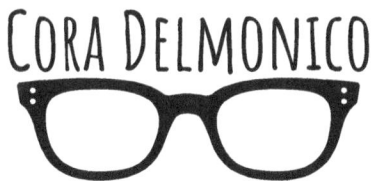

TIP: USE CRAYONS, COLORED PENCILS, OR GEL PENS.
IF YOU WANT TO USE MARKERS, PUT A SHEET OF PAPER BETWEEN PAGES
TO ELIMINATE BLEED THROUGH.

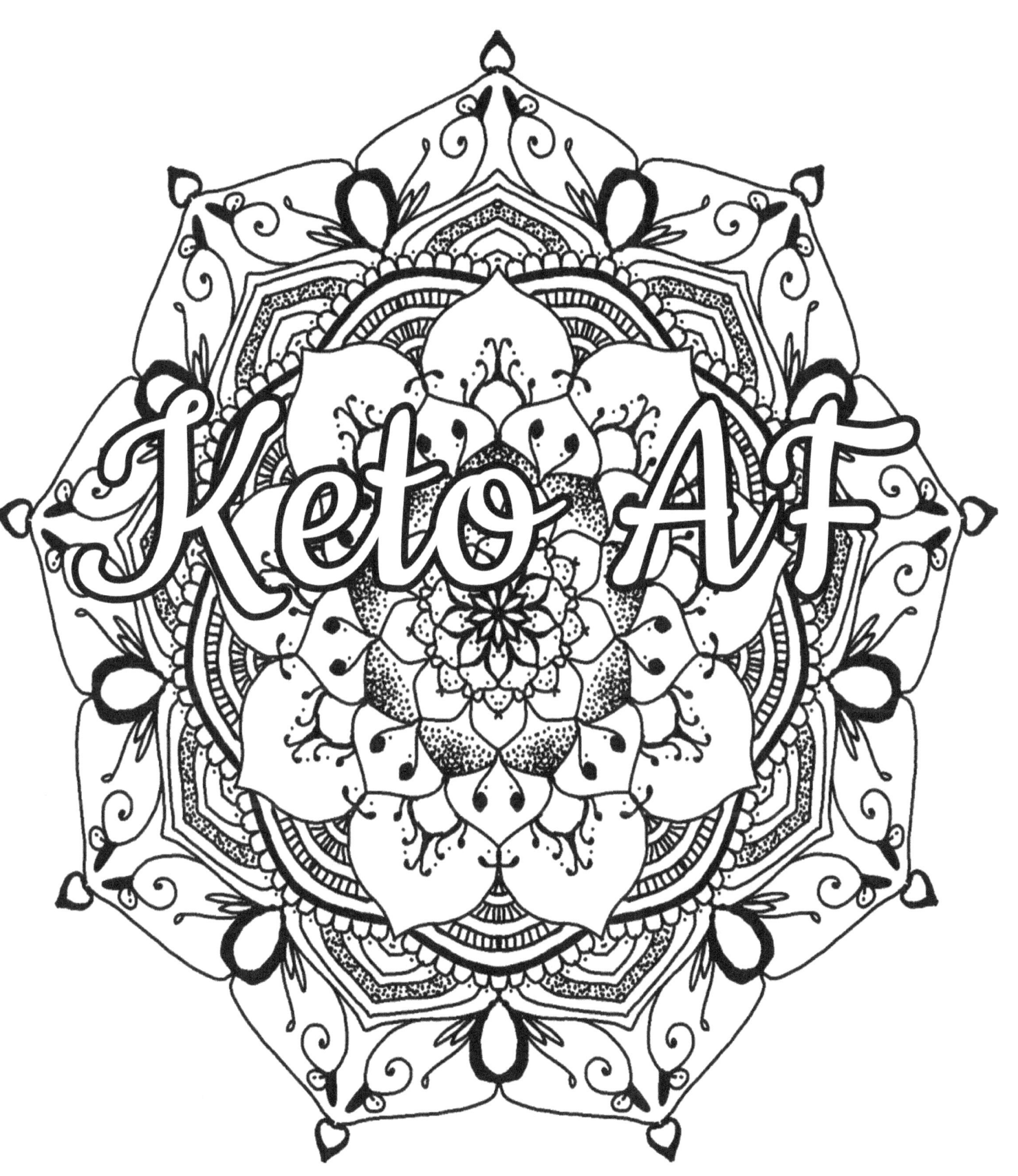

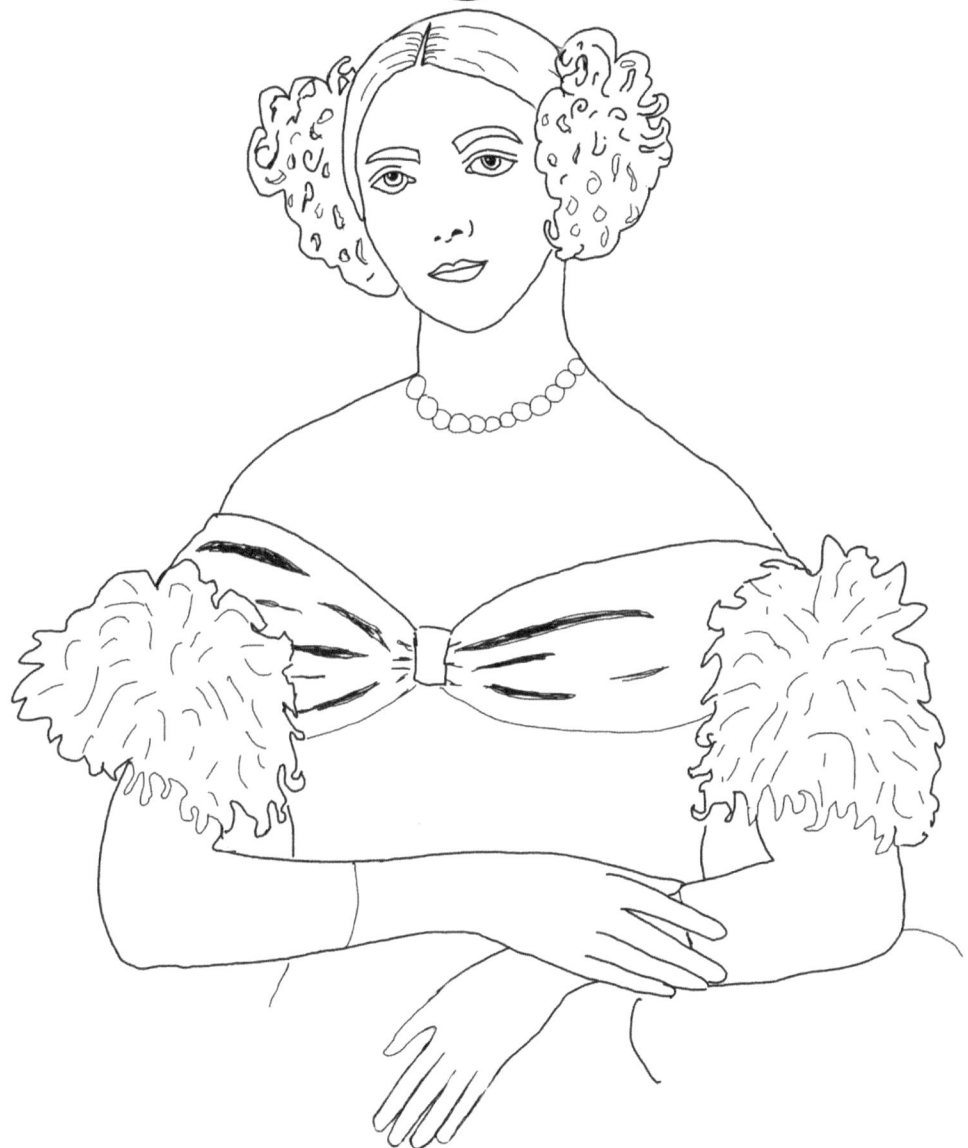

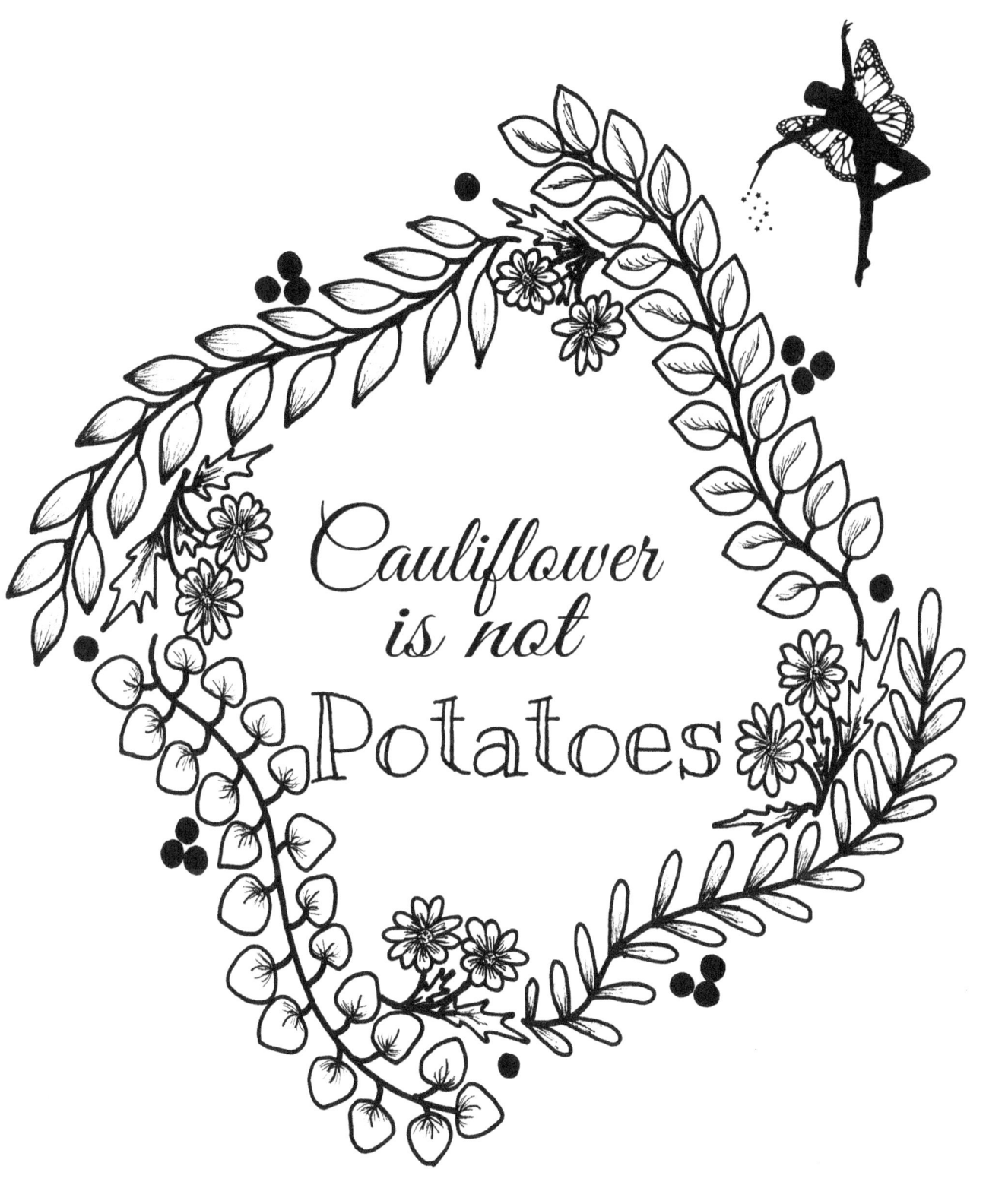

Lost 2 Pounds!

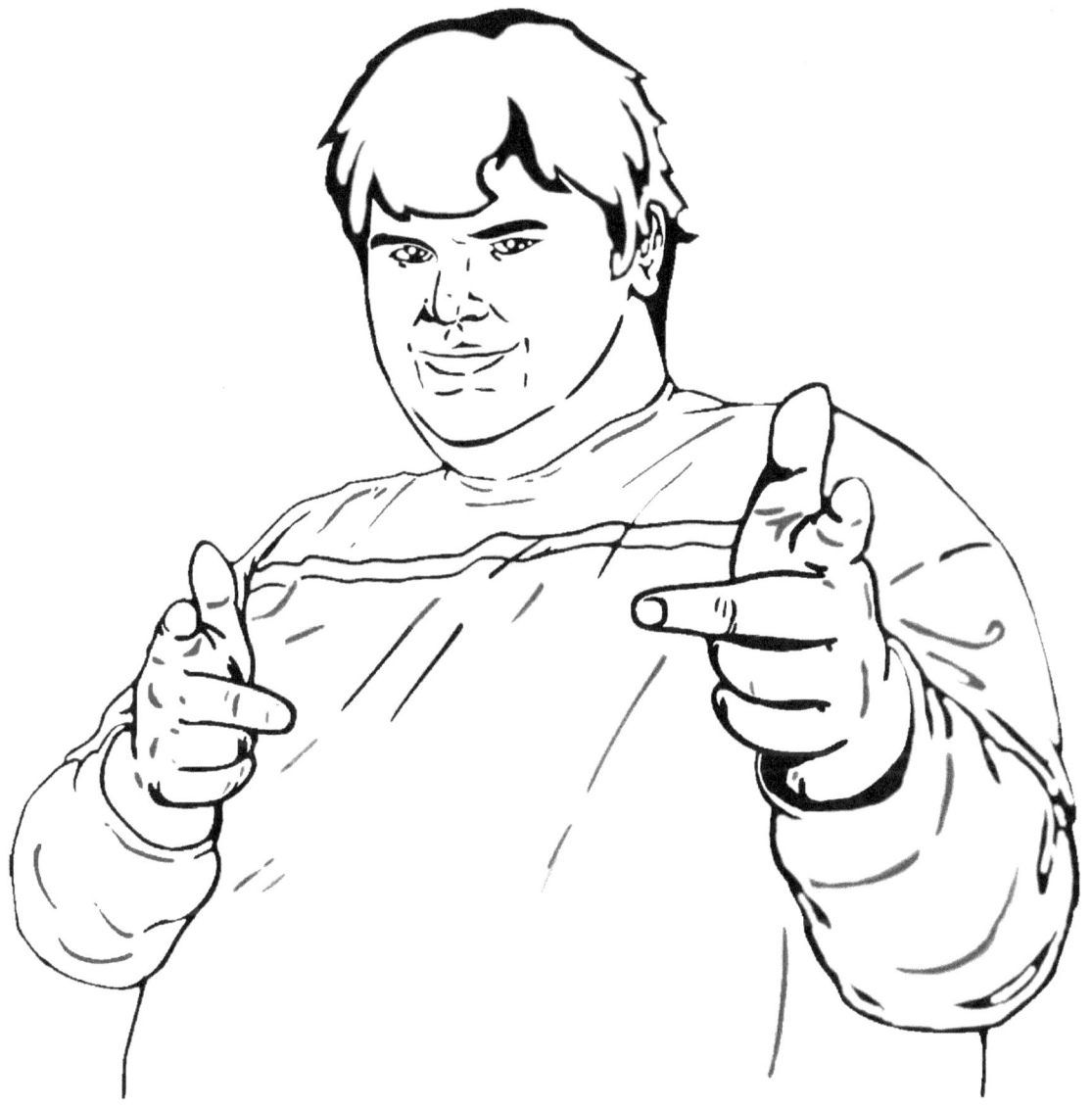

Rewarding myself with

A CHEESEBURGER...

NOT ONLY DID I FALL OFF THE DIET WAGON,

I dragged it into the woods,

SET IT ON FIRE,

and used the insurance money

to buy cupcakes!

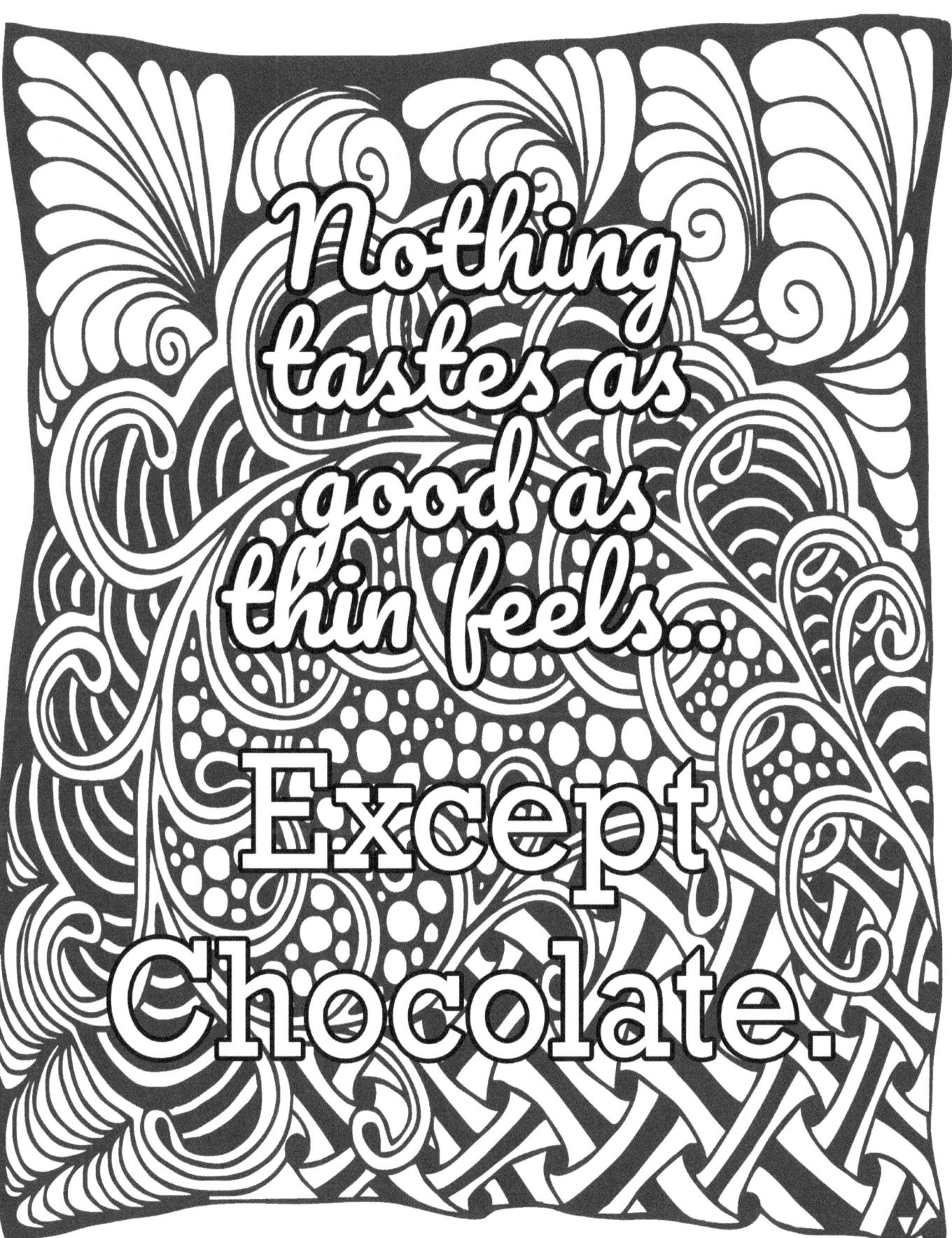

When I am still hungry & out of macros...

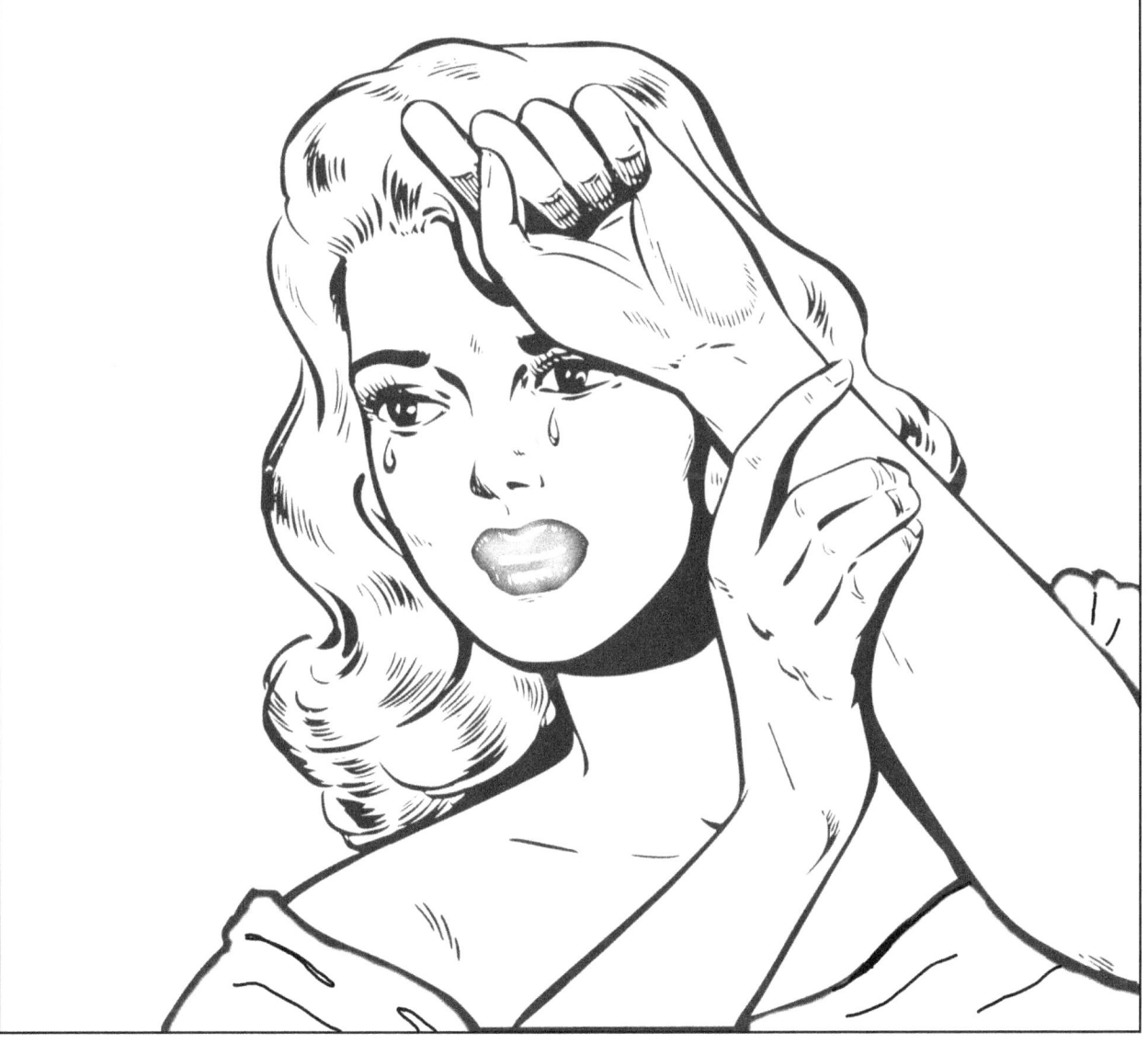

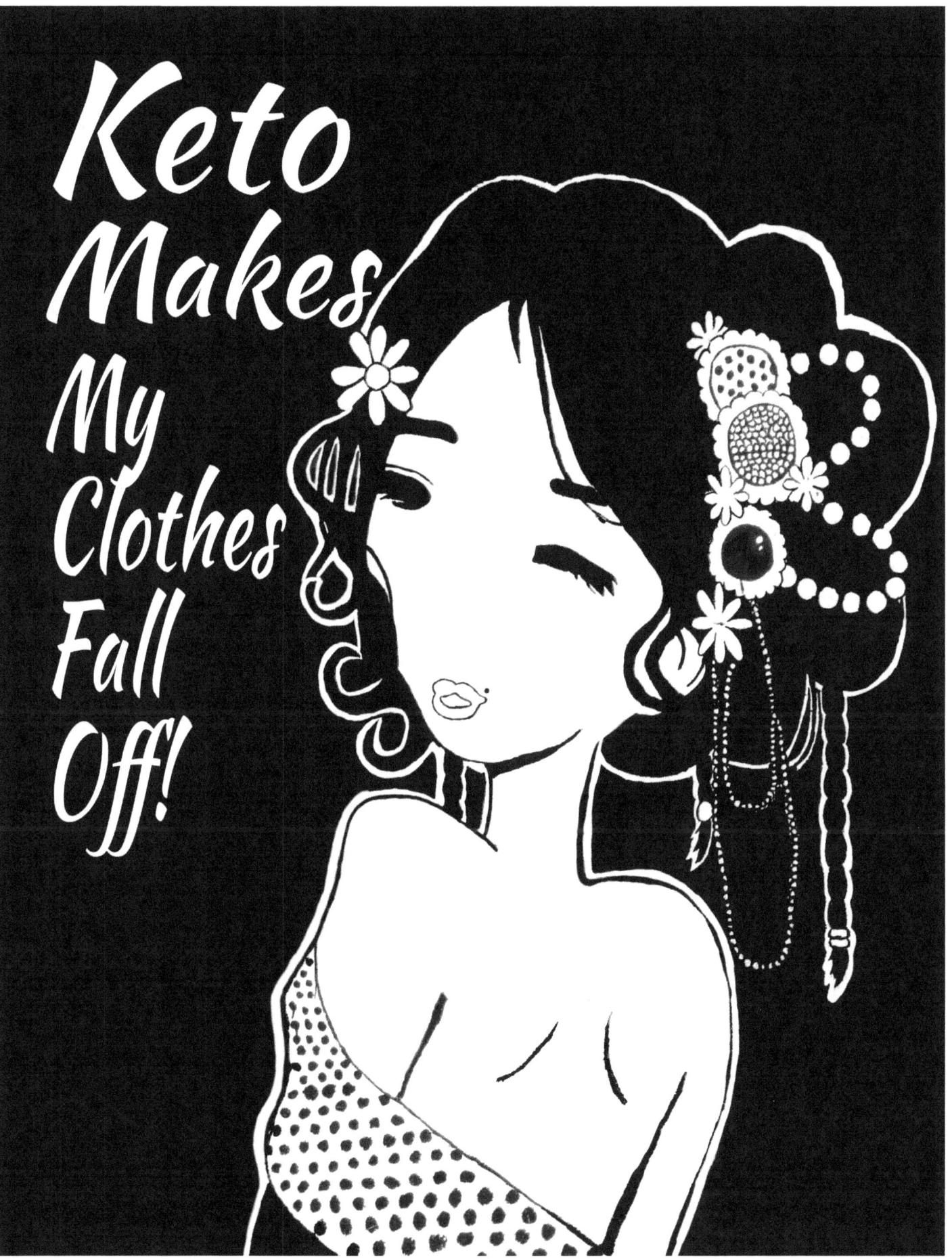

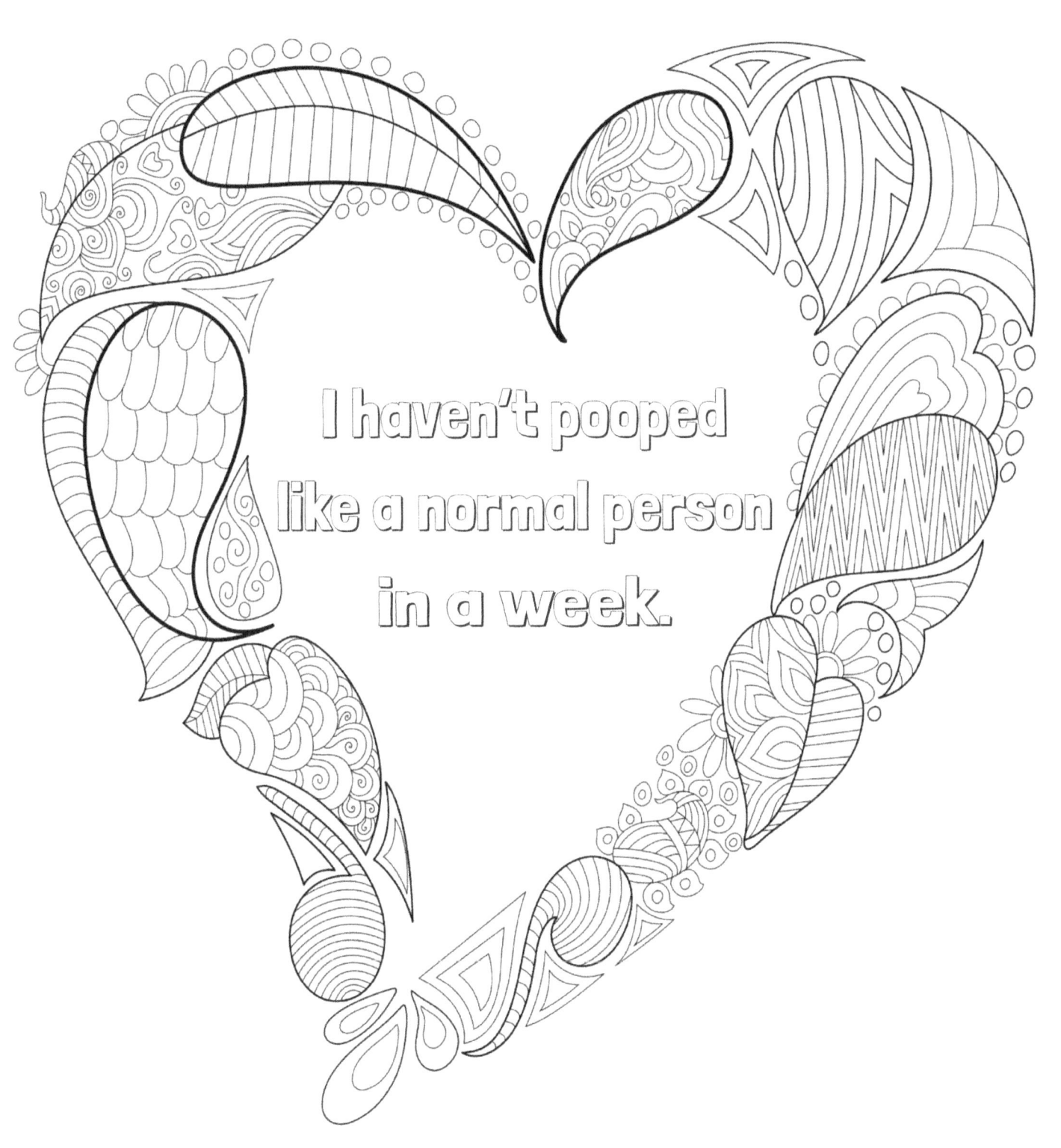

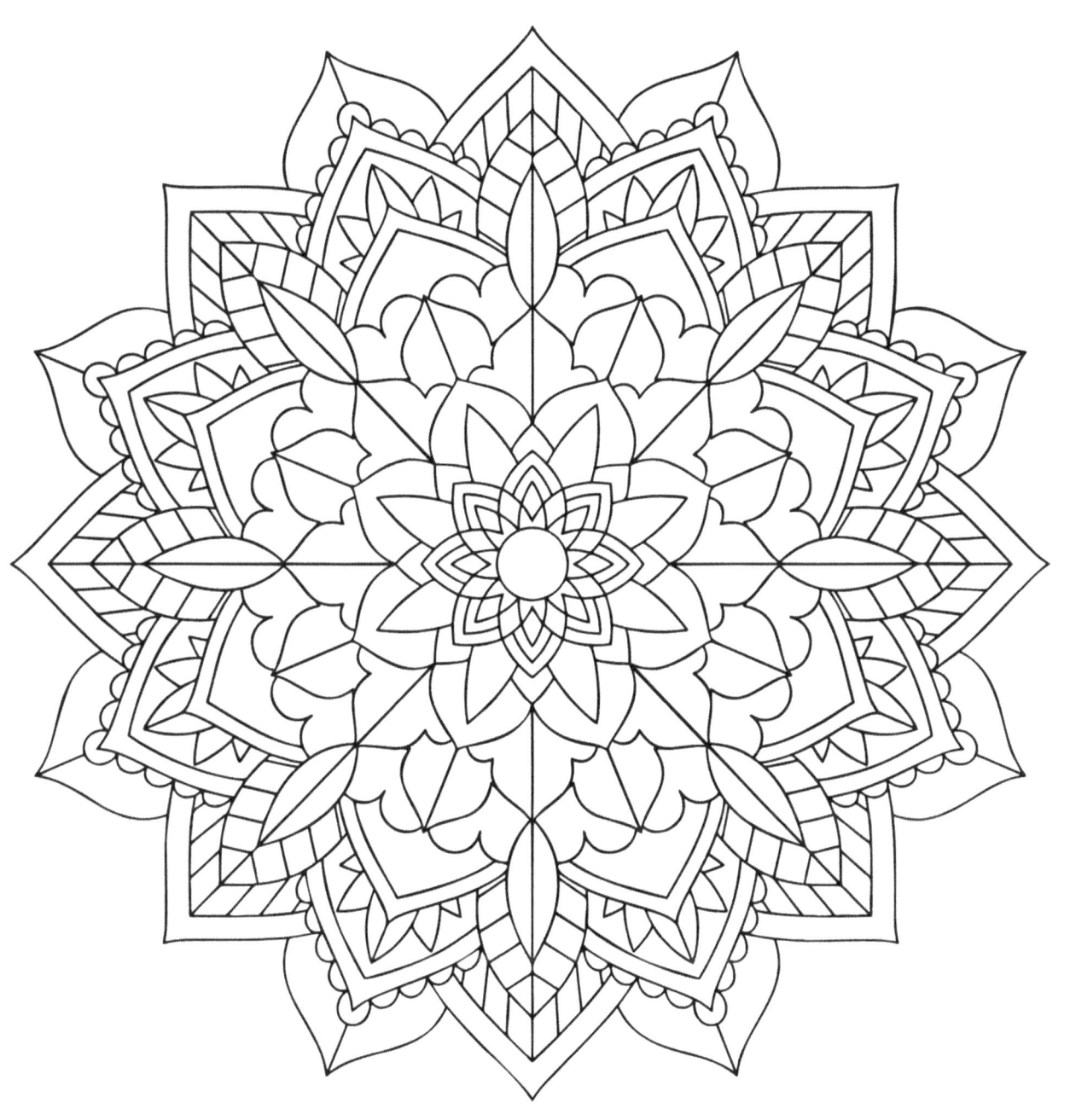

I JUST WANT
A COOKIE

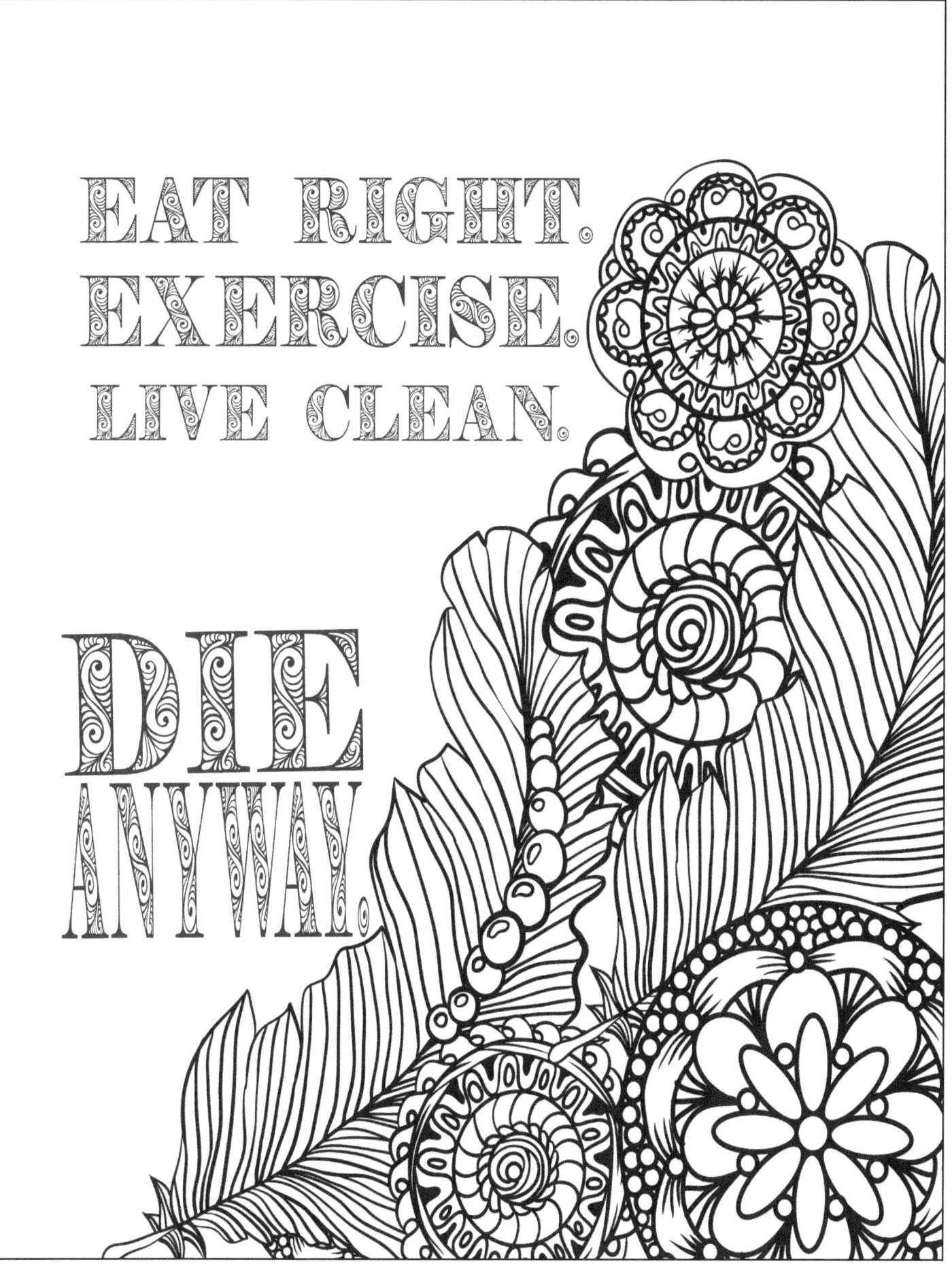

I would lose weight but

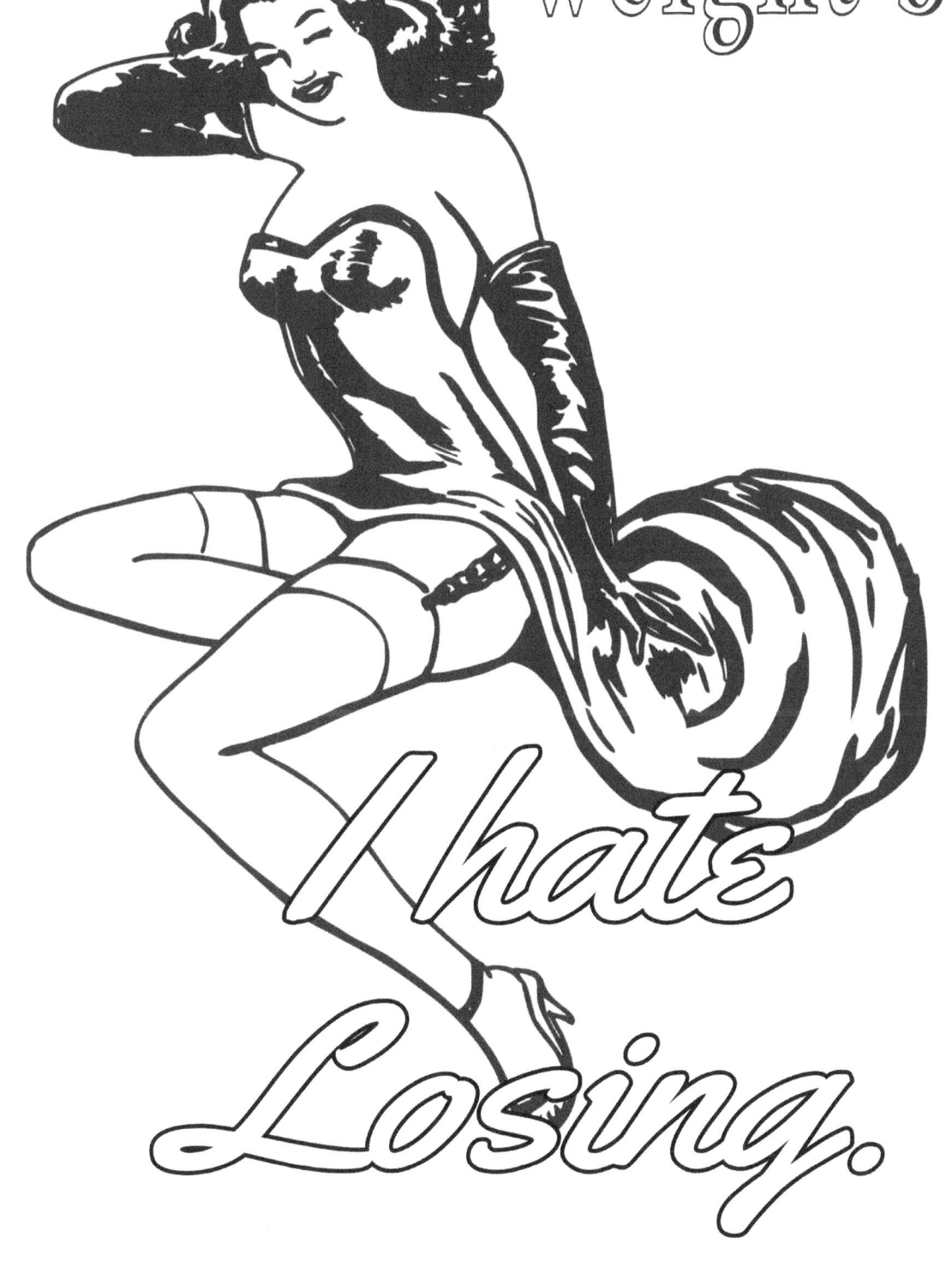

I hate Losing.

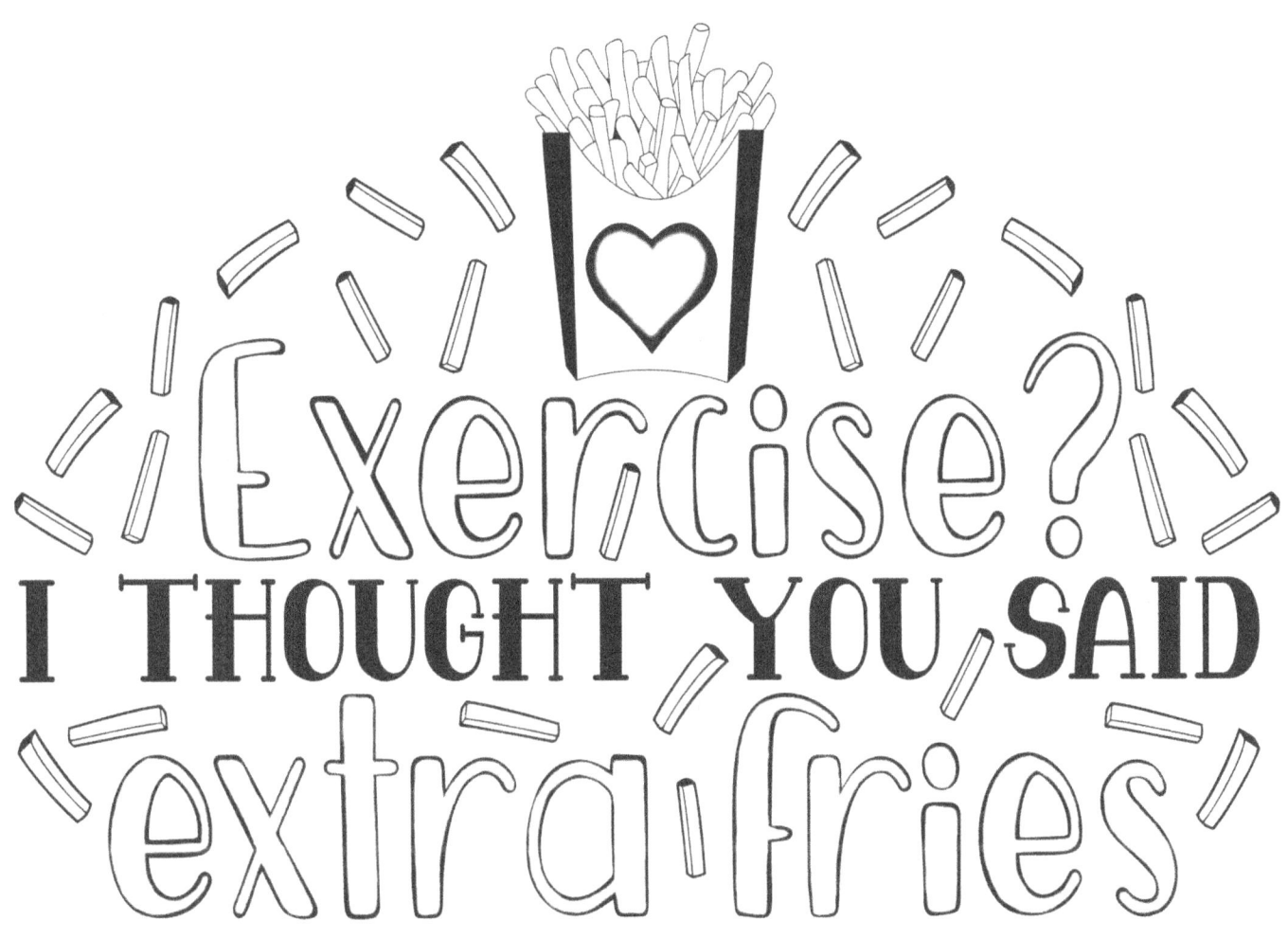

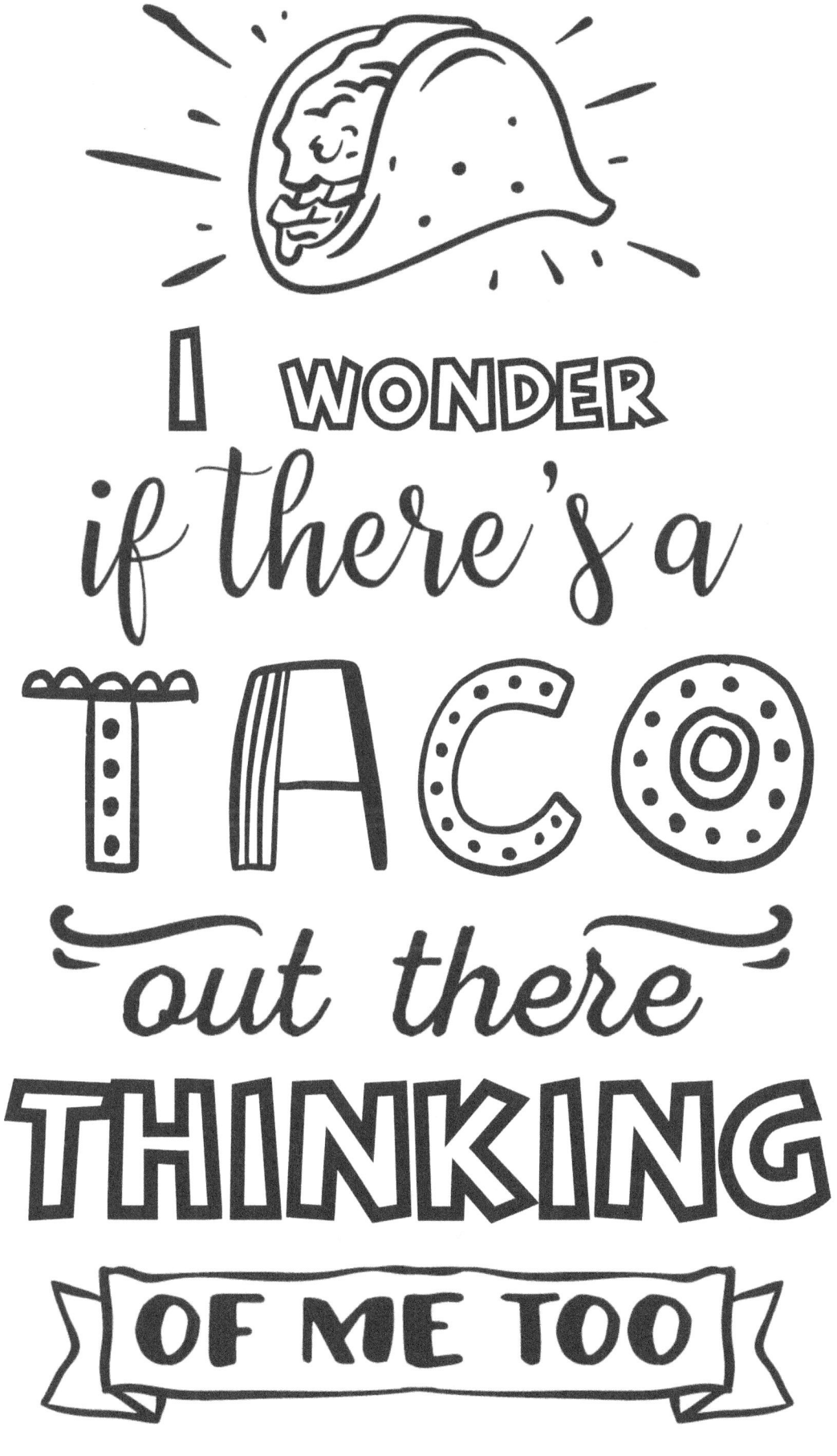

I WONDER if there's a TACO out there THINKING OF ME TOO

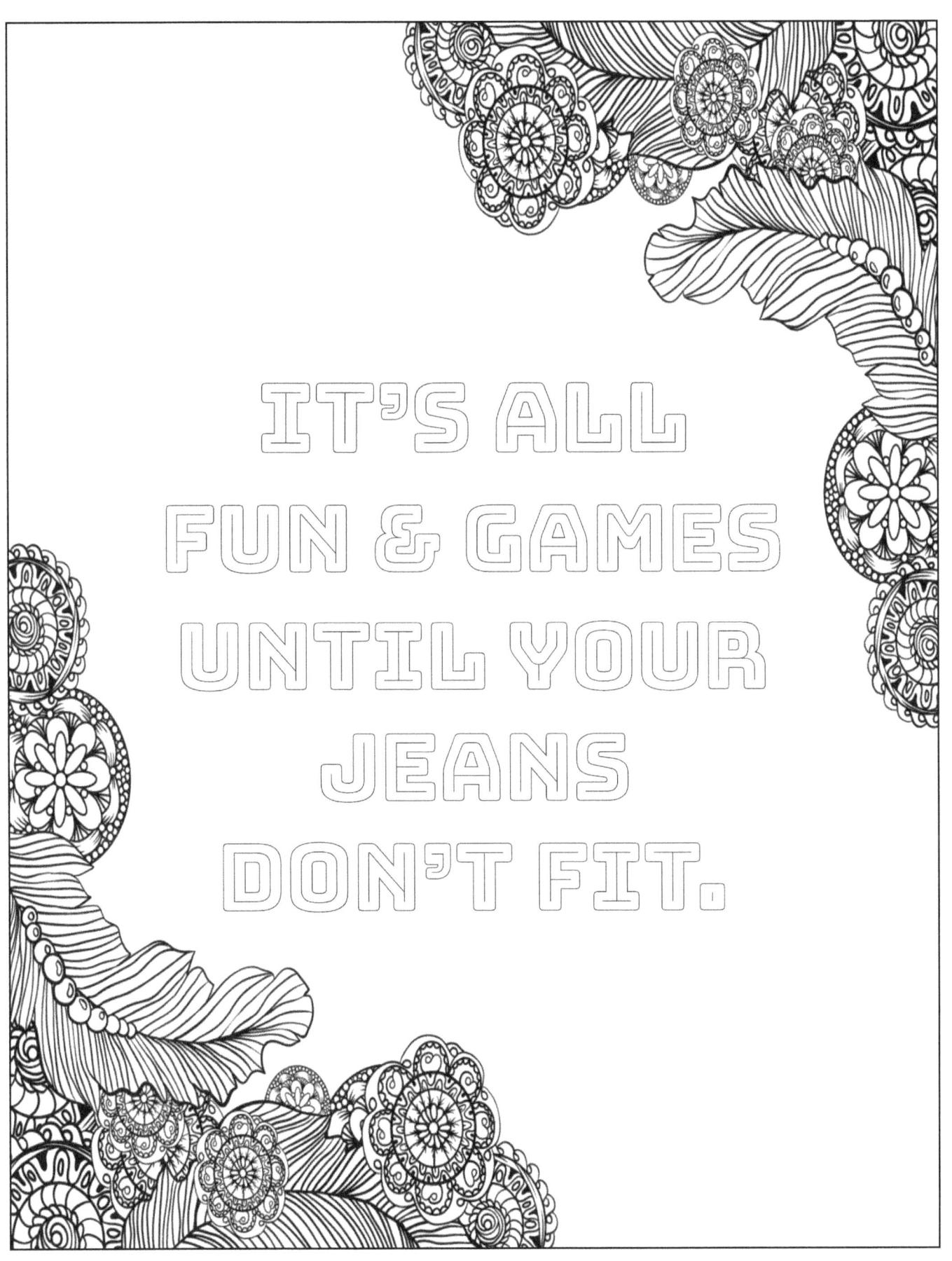

IT'S ALL
FUN & GAMES
UNTIL YOUR
JEANS
DON'T FIT.

BACON MAKES EVERYTHING BETTER

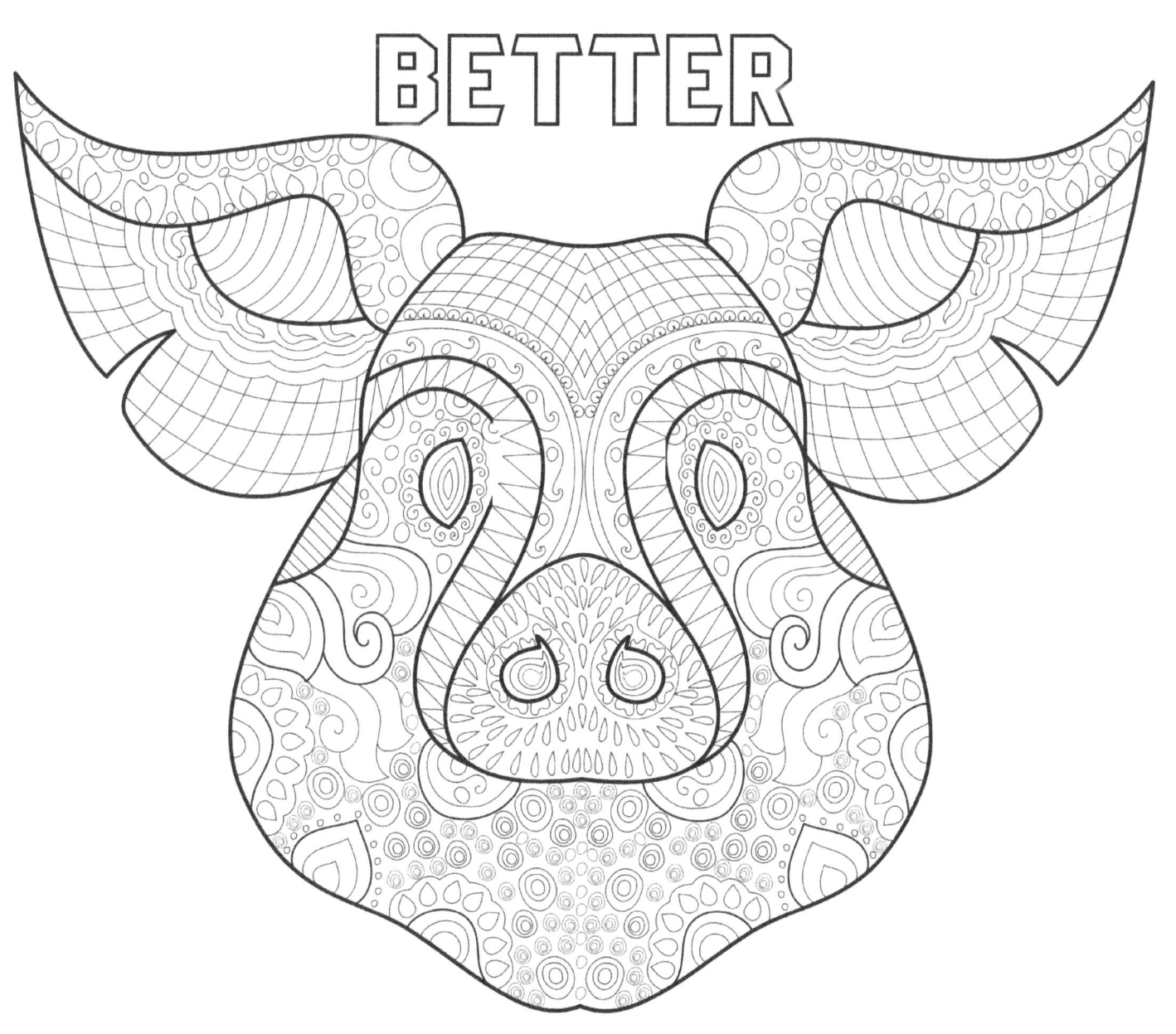

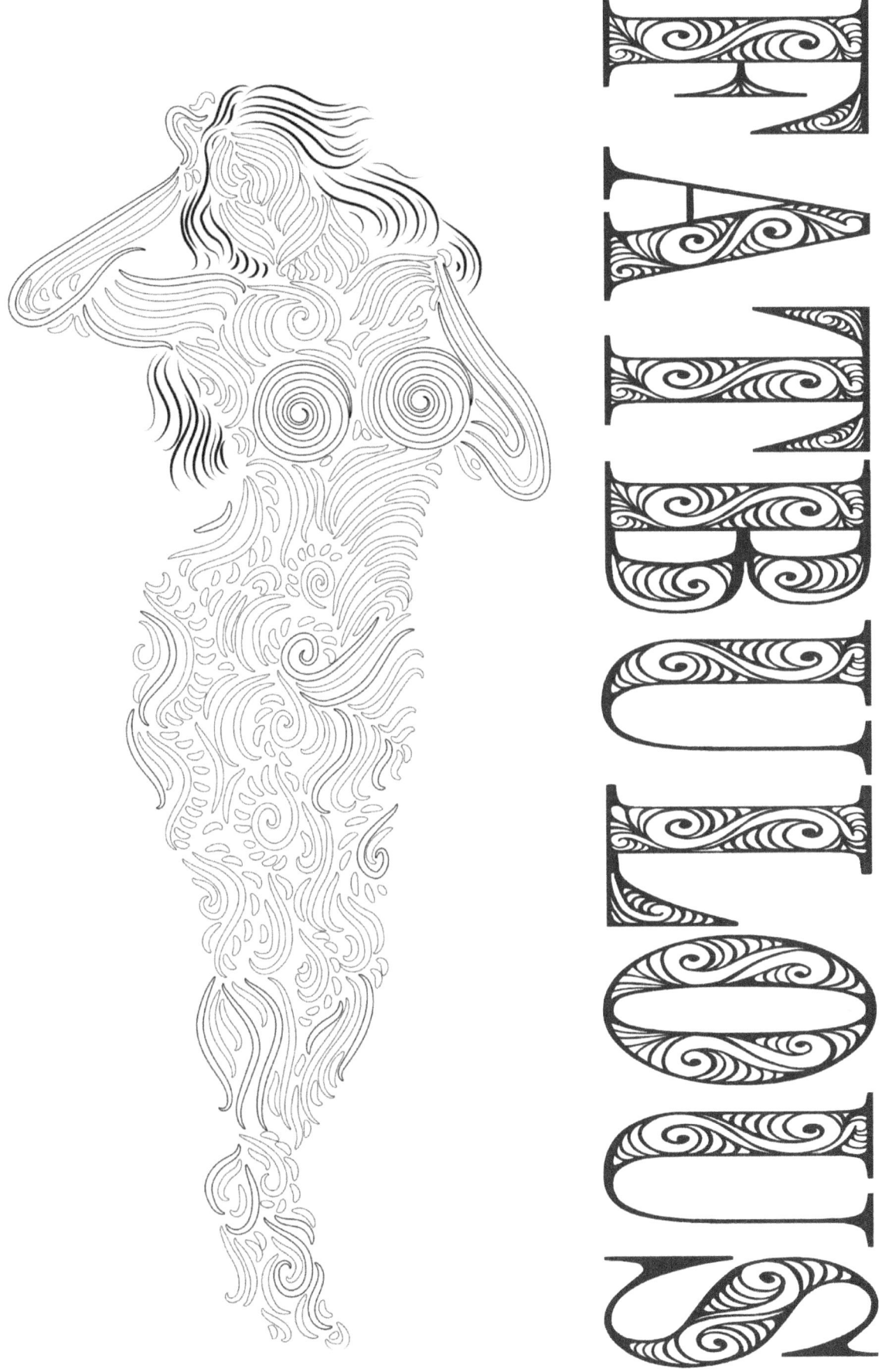

RANGITOTO

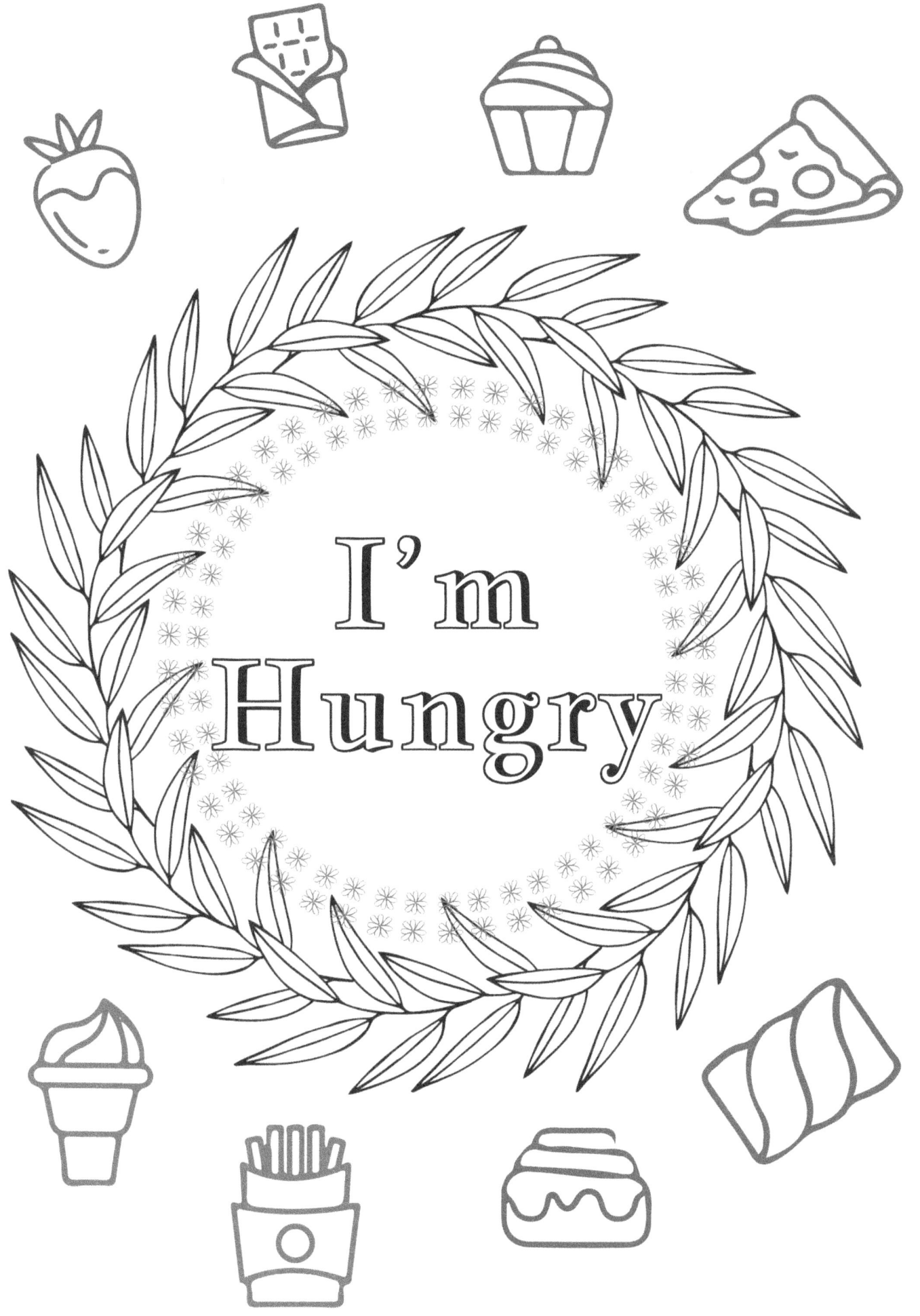

I'M NOT FAT

I'm just

EASY TO See!

I'm in shape.
Round is a shape.

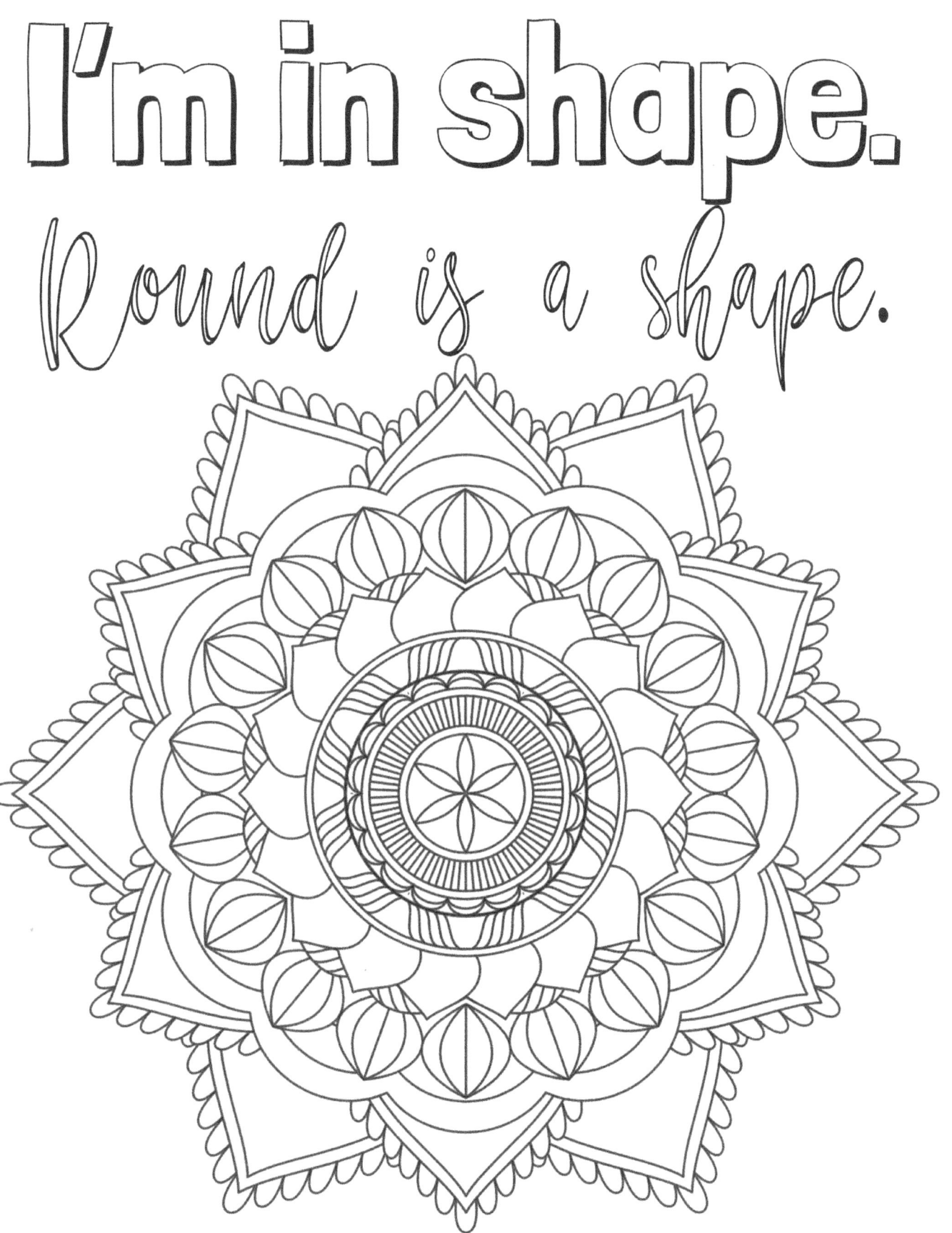

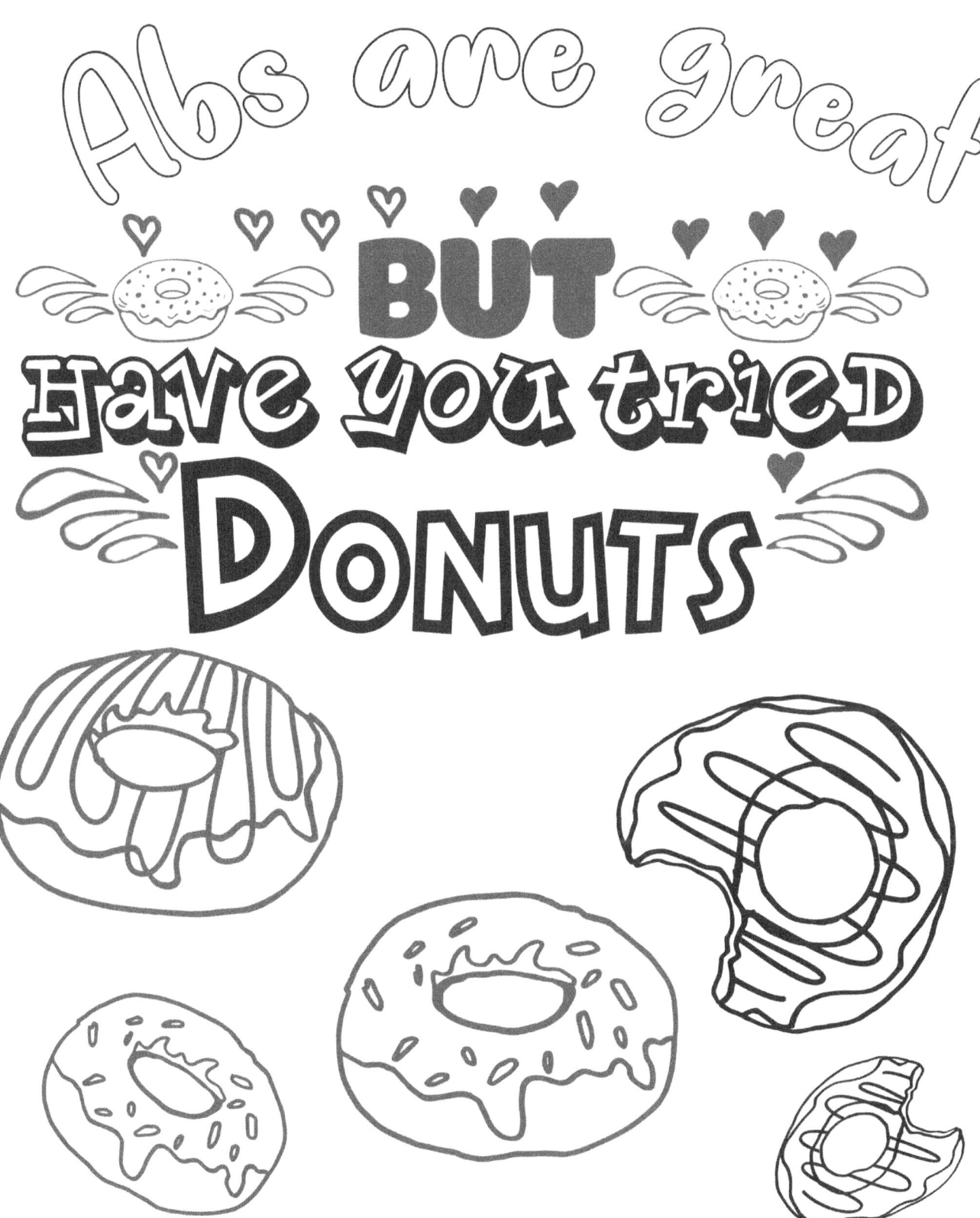

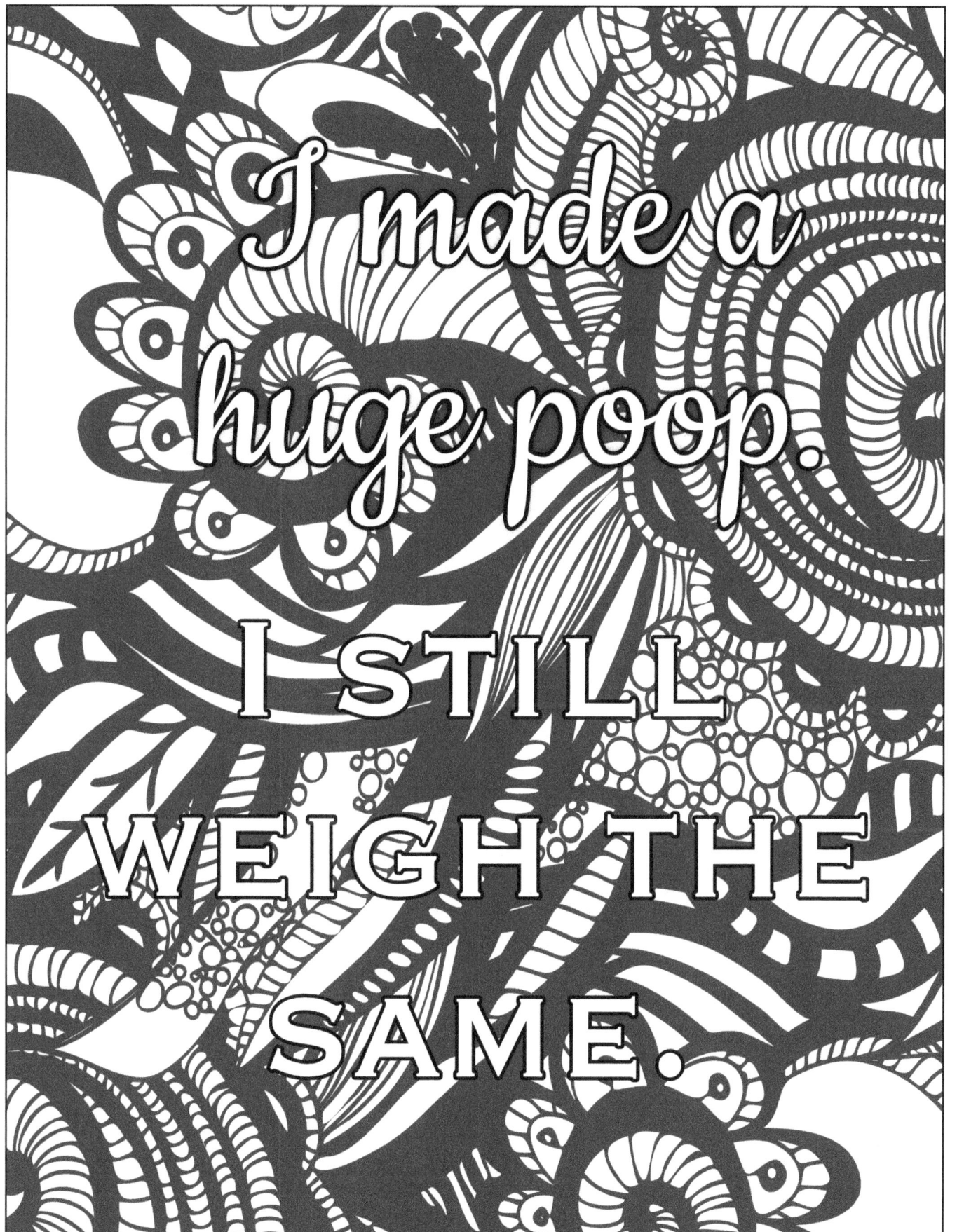

Chocolate Doesn't Ask Silly Questions.

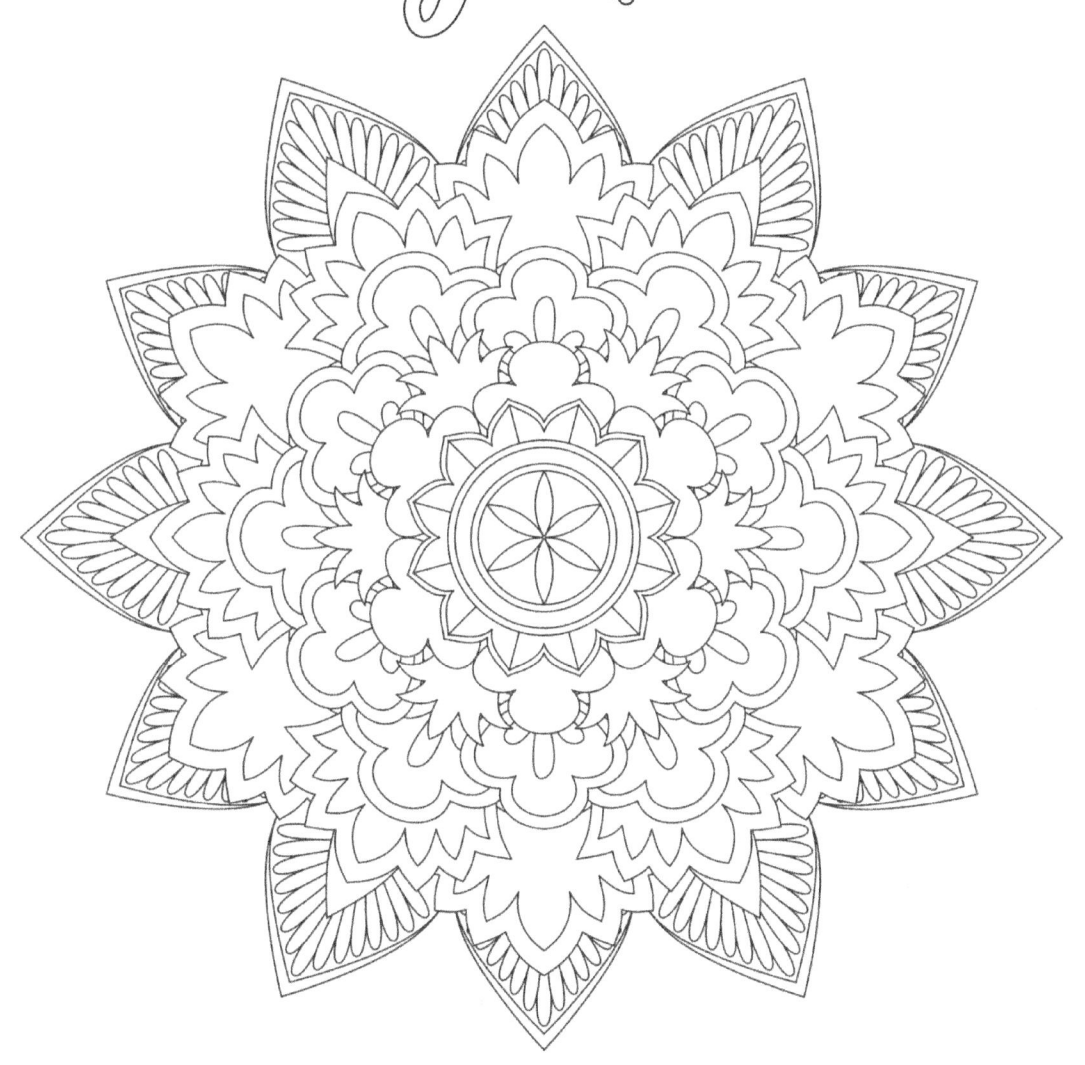

CHOCOLATE UNDERSTANDS

I WANT TO LOSE WEIGHT.

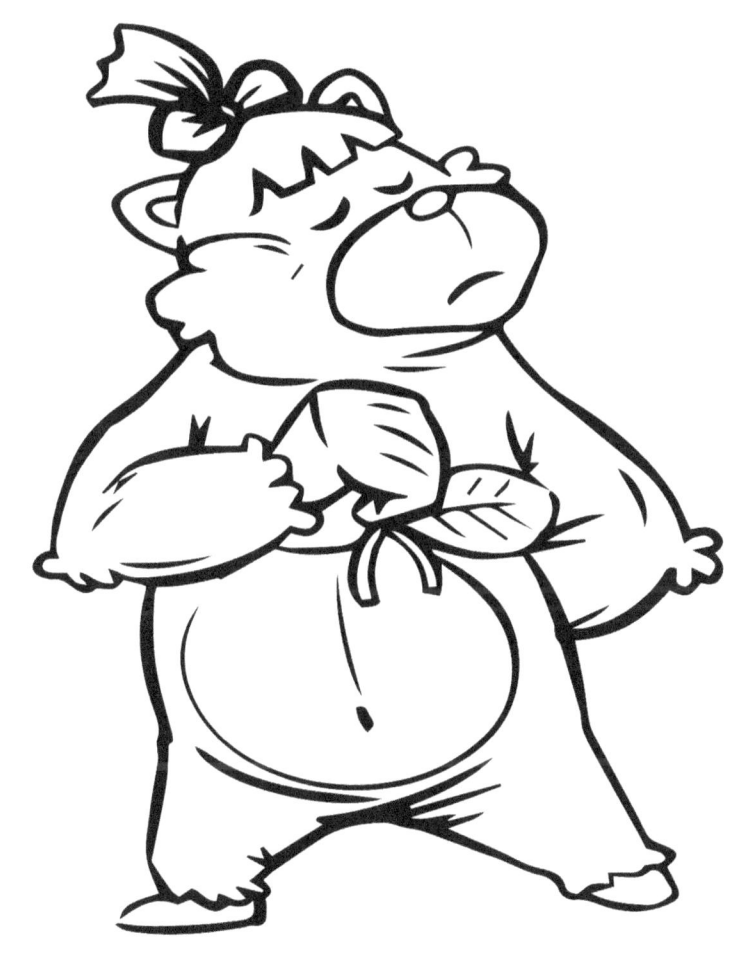

My weight doesn't want to lose me!

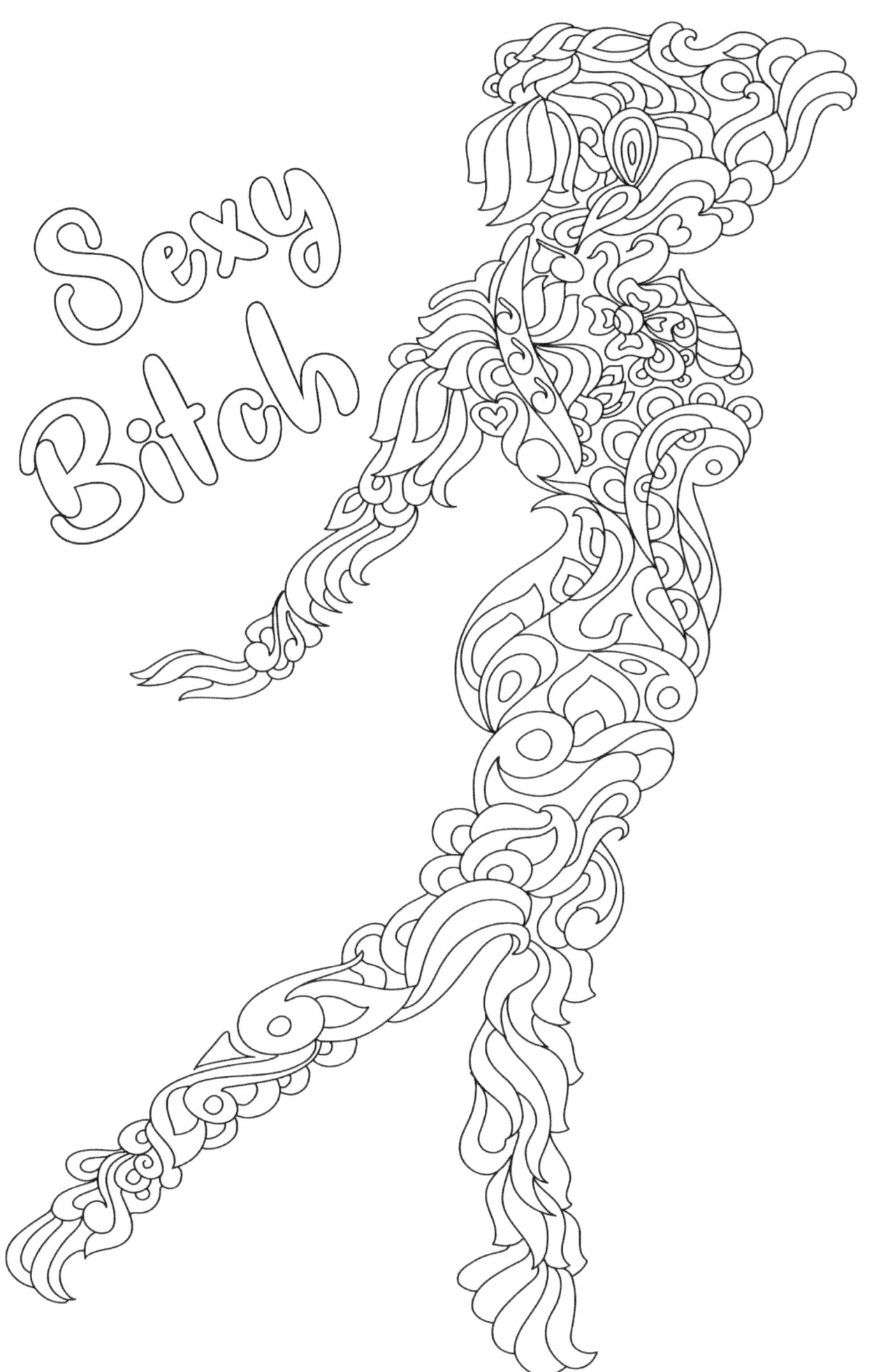

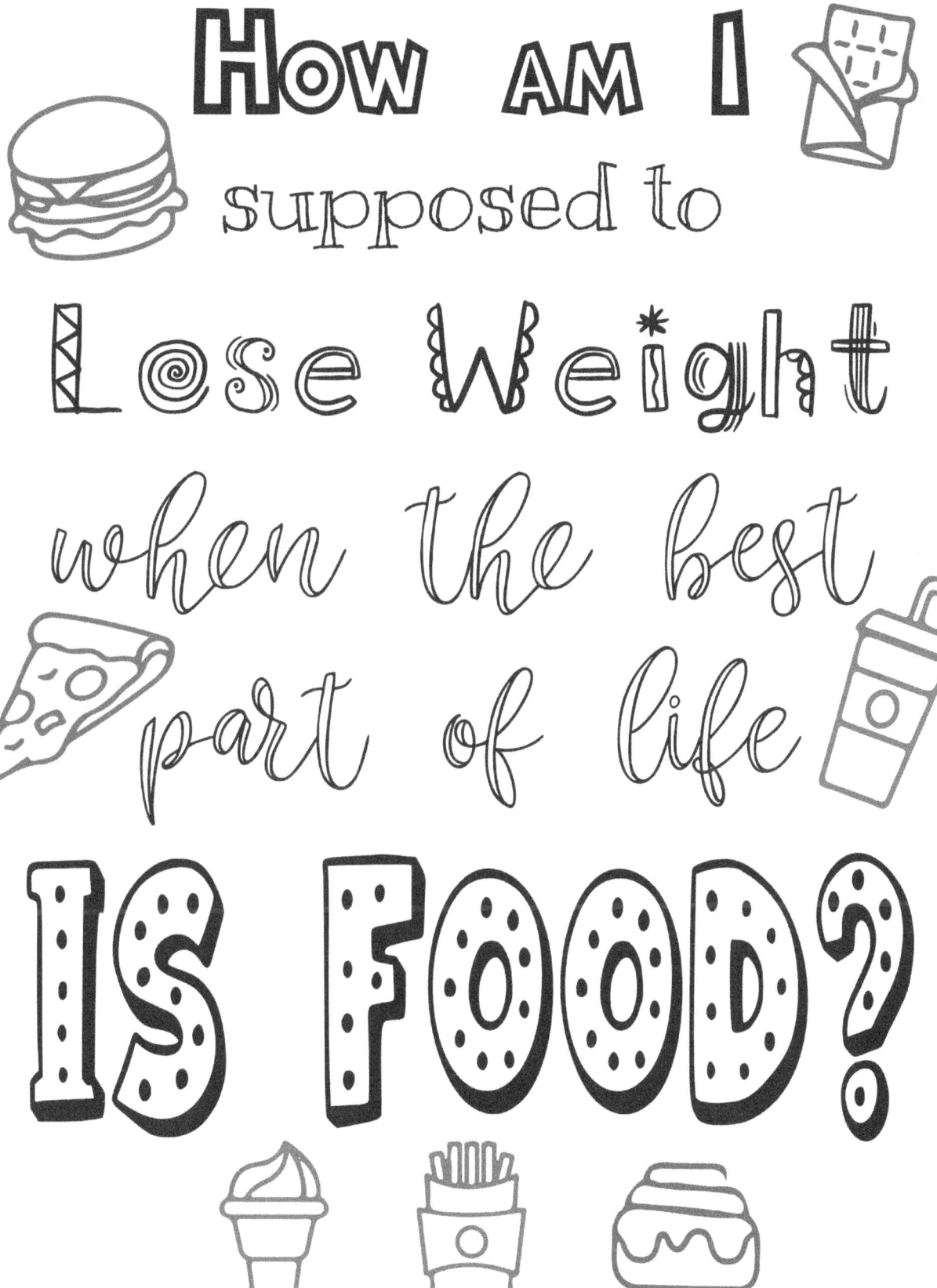

How am I supposed to Lose Weight when the best part of life IS FOOD?

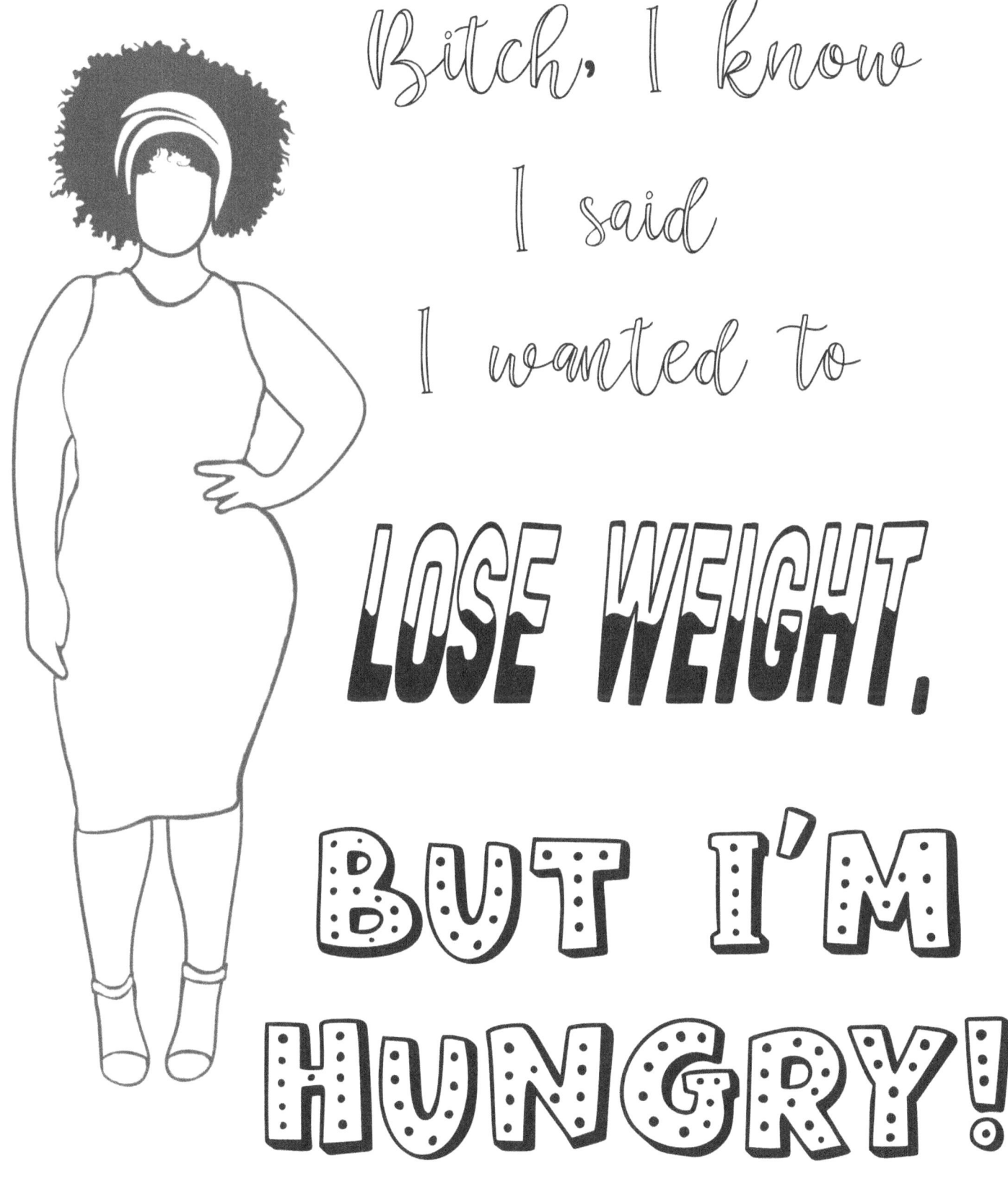

Diet Tip:

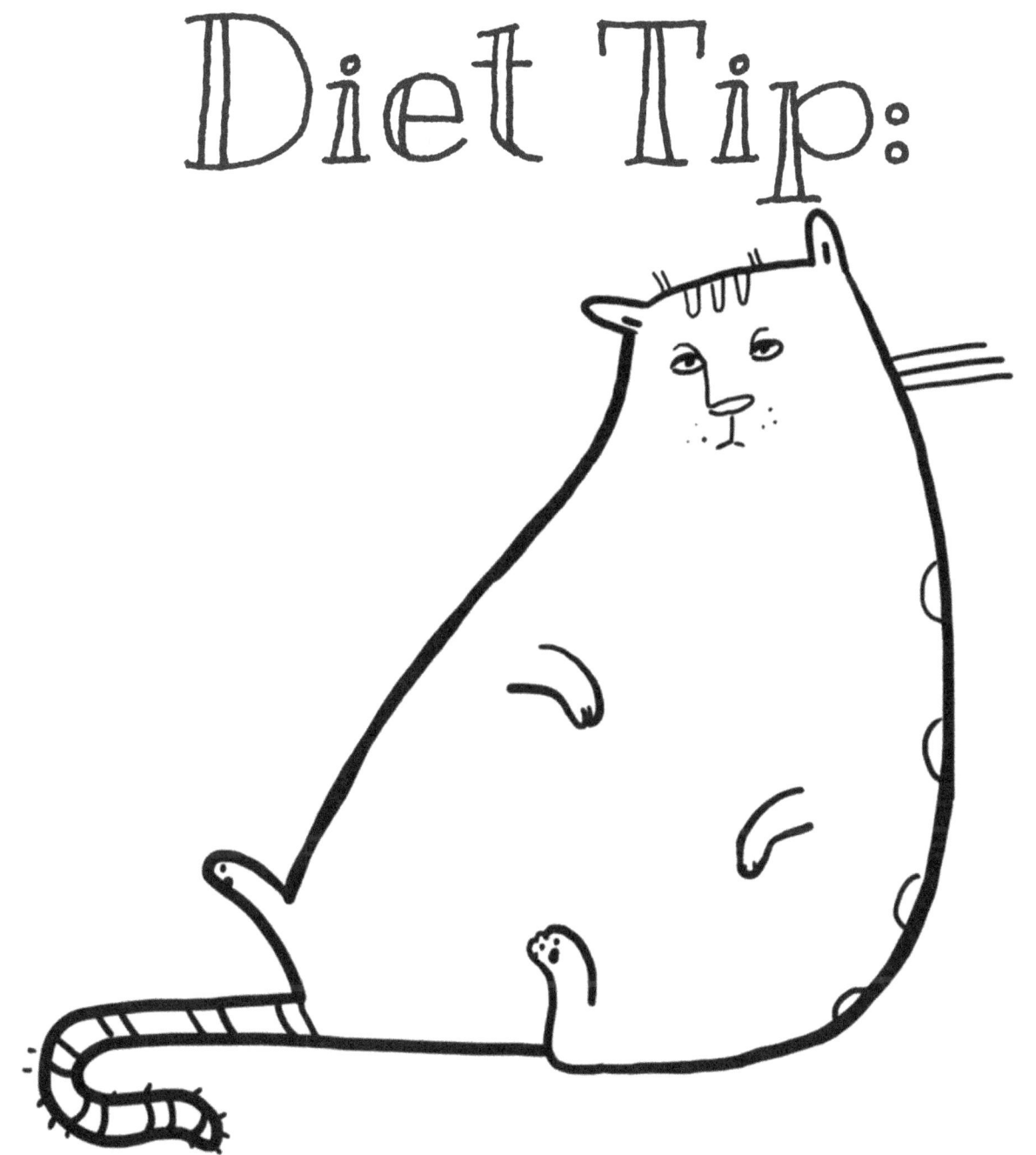

Spend your paycheck on shoes & spas
and you won't have money
for food.

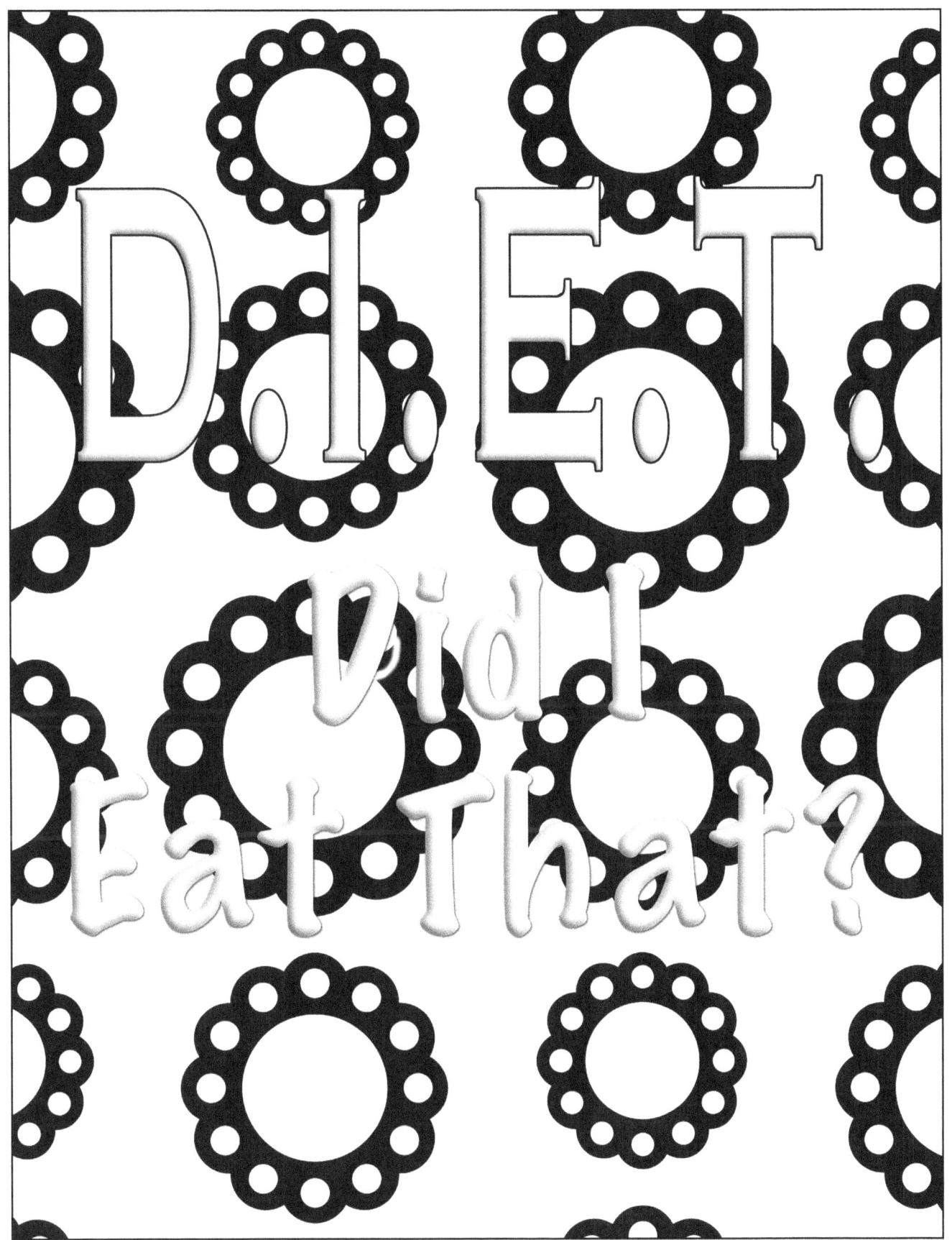

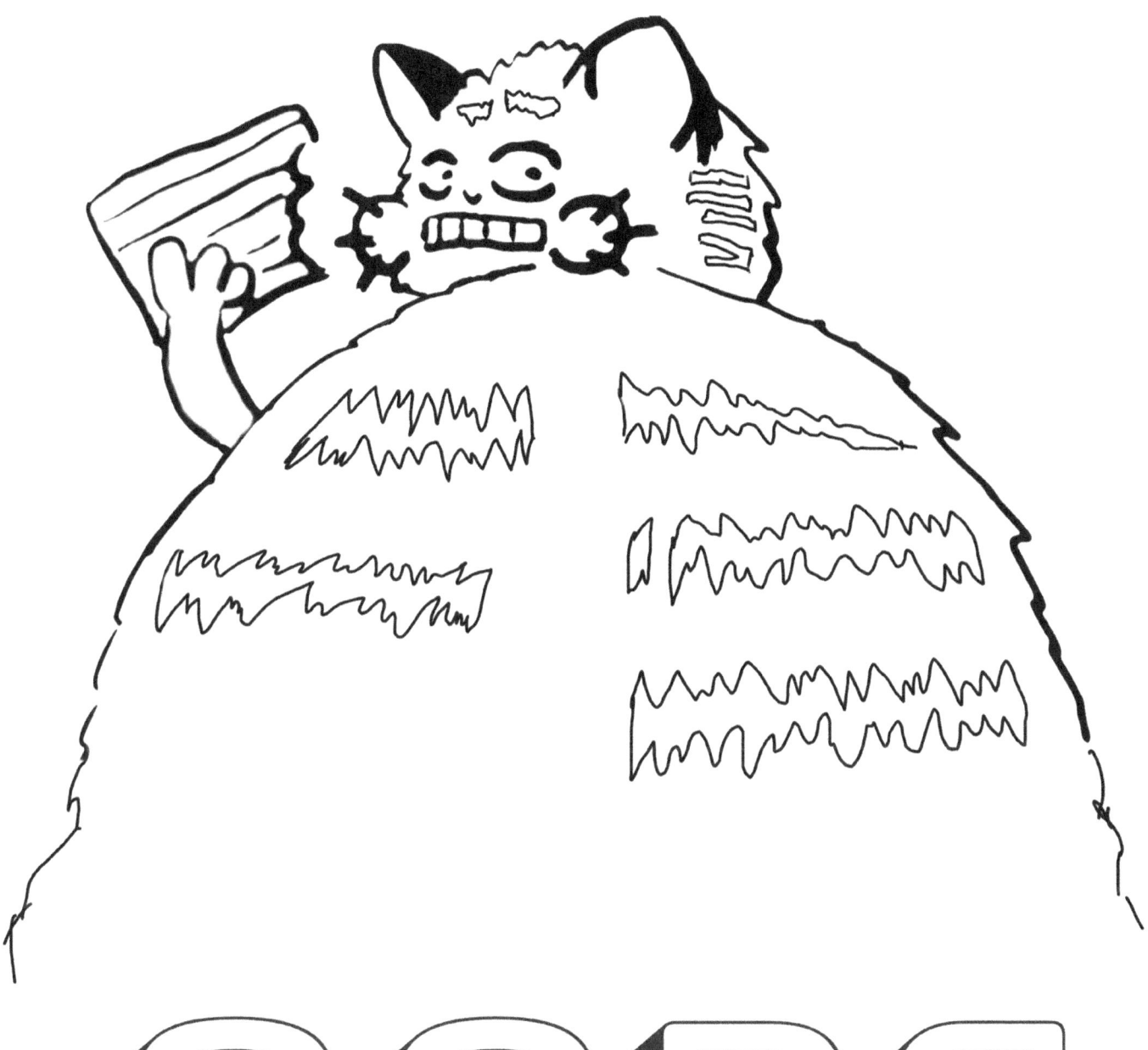

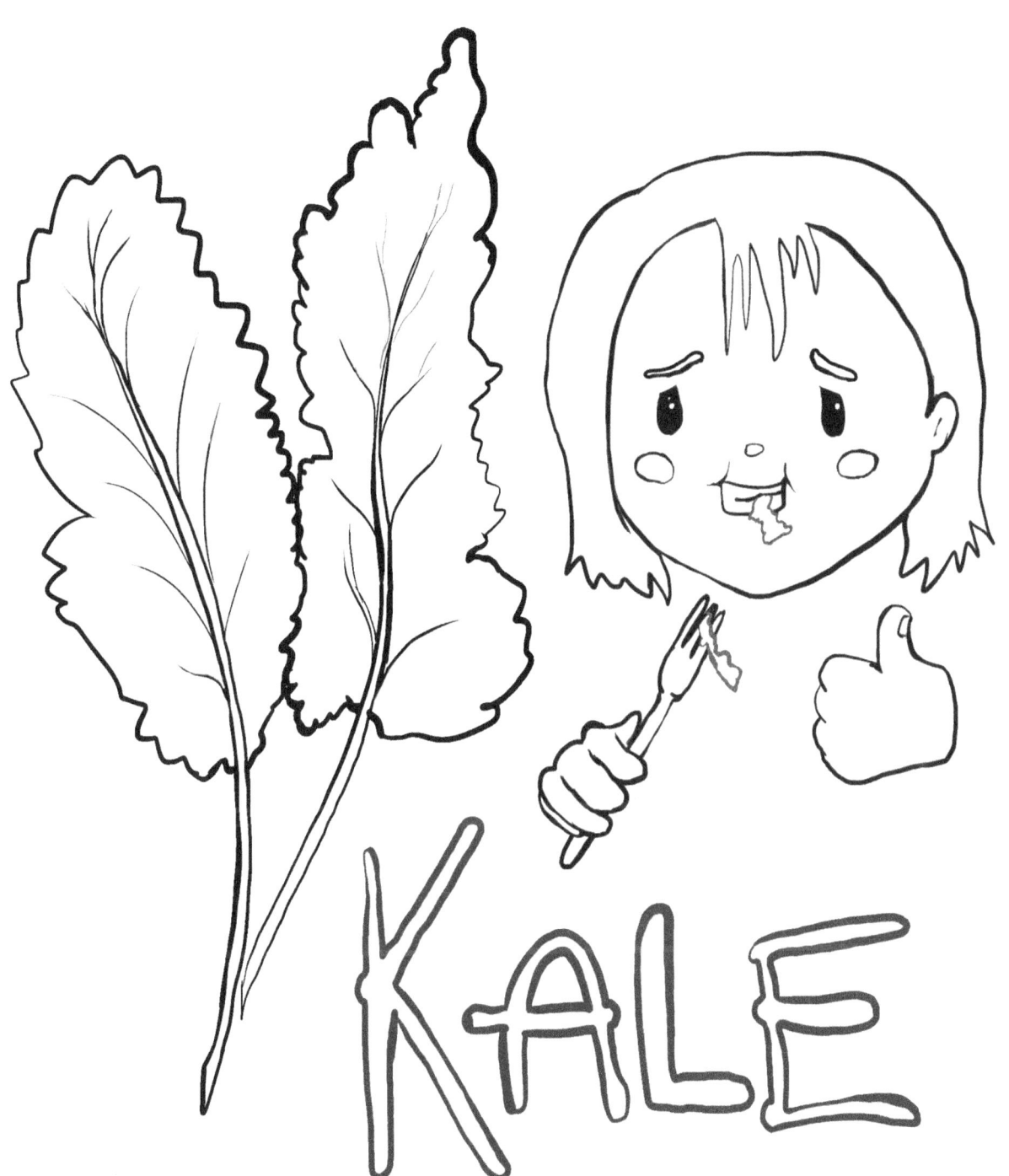

KALE

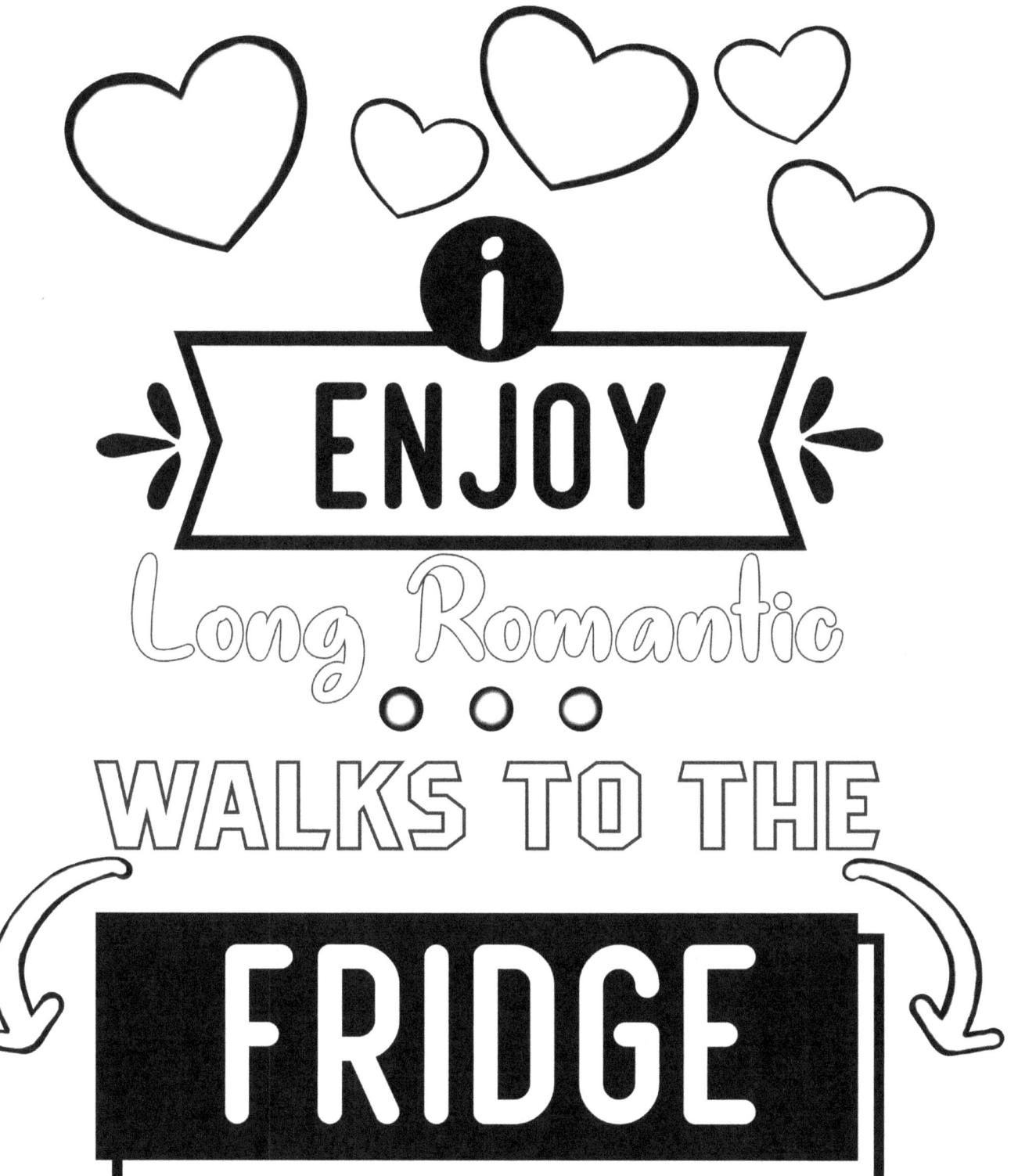

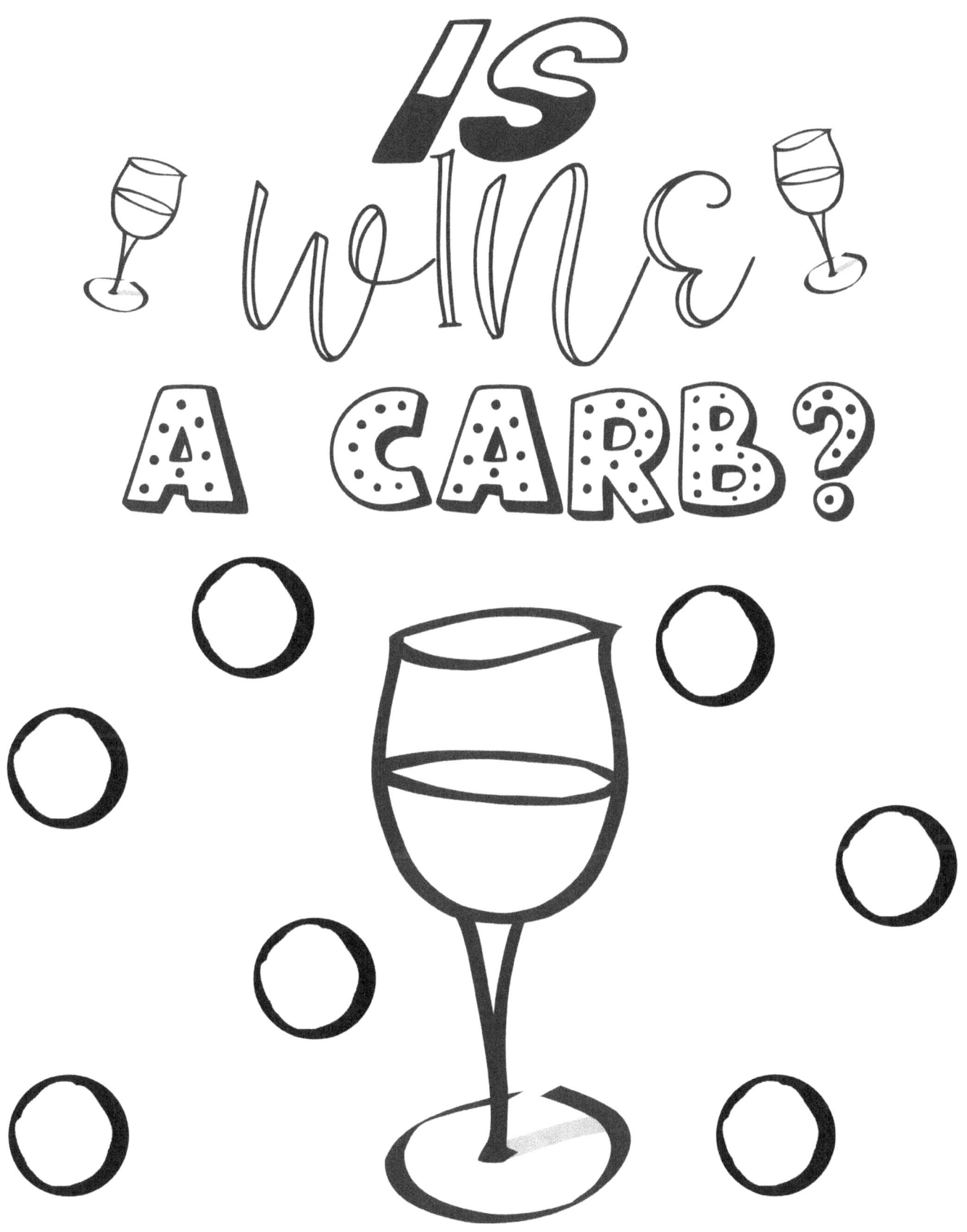

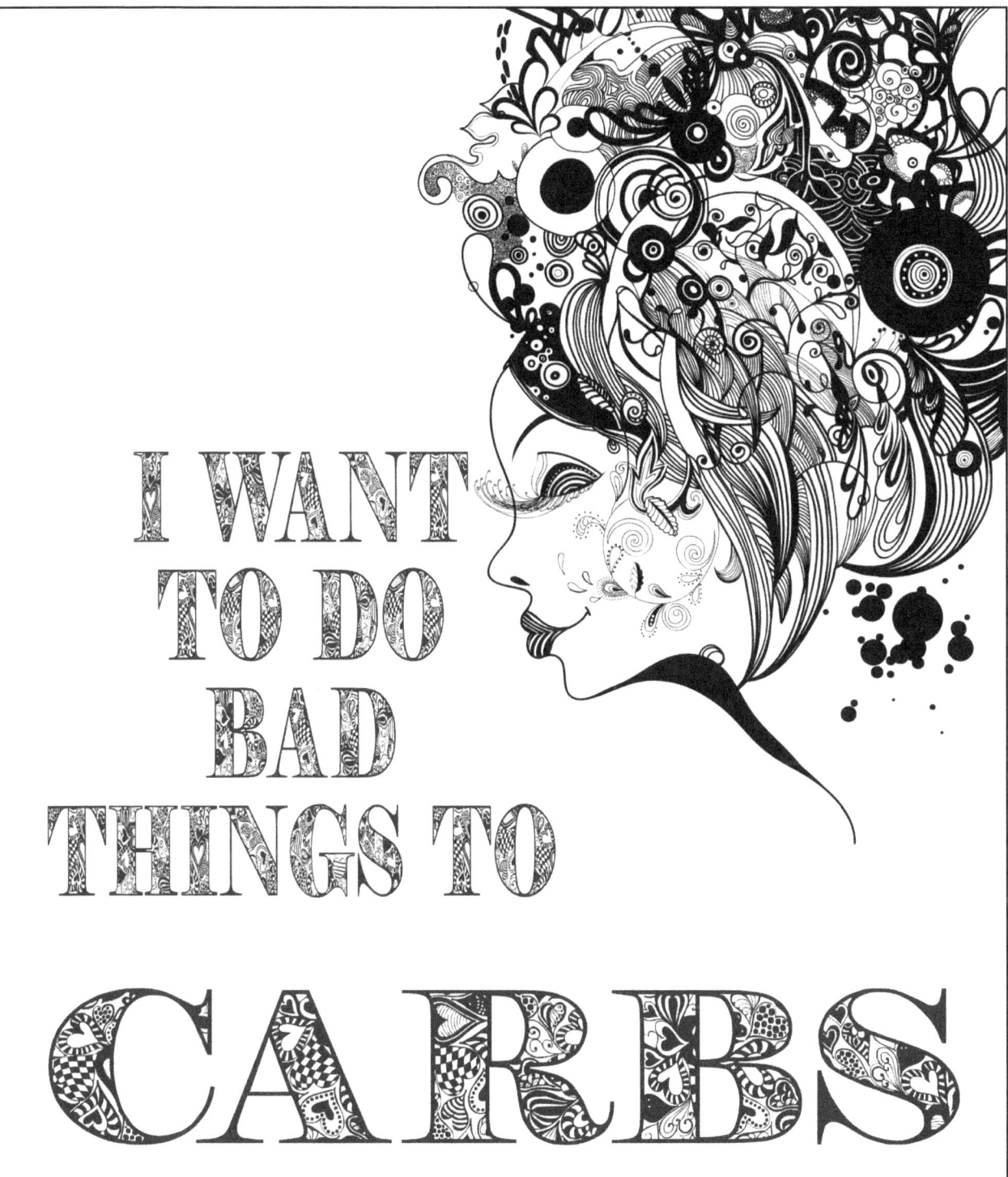

I WANT
TO DO
BAD
THINGS TO
CARBS

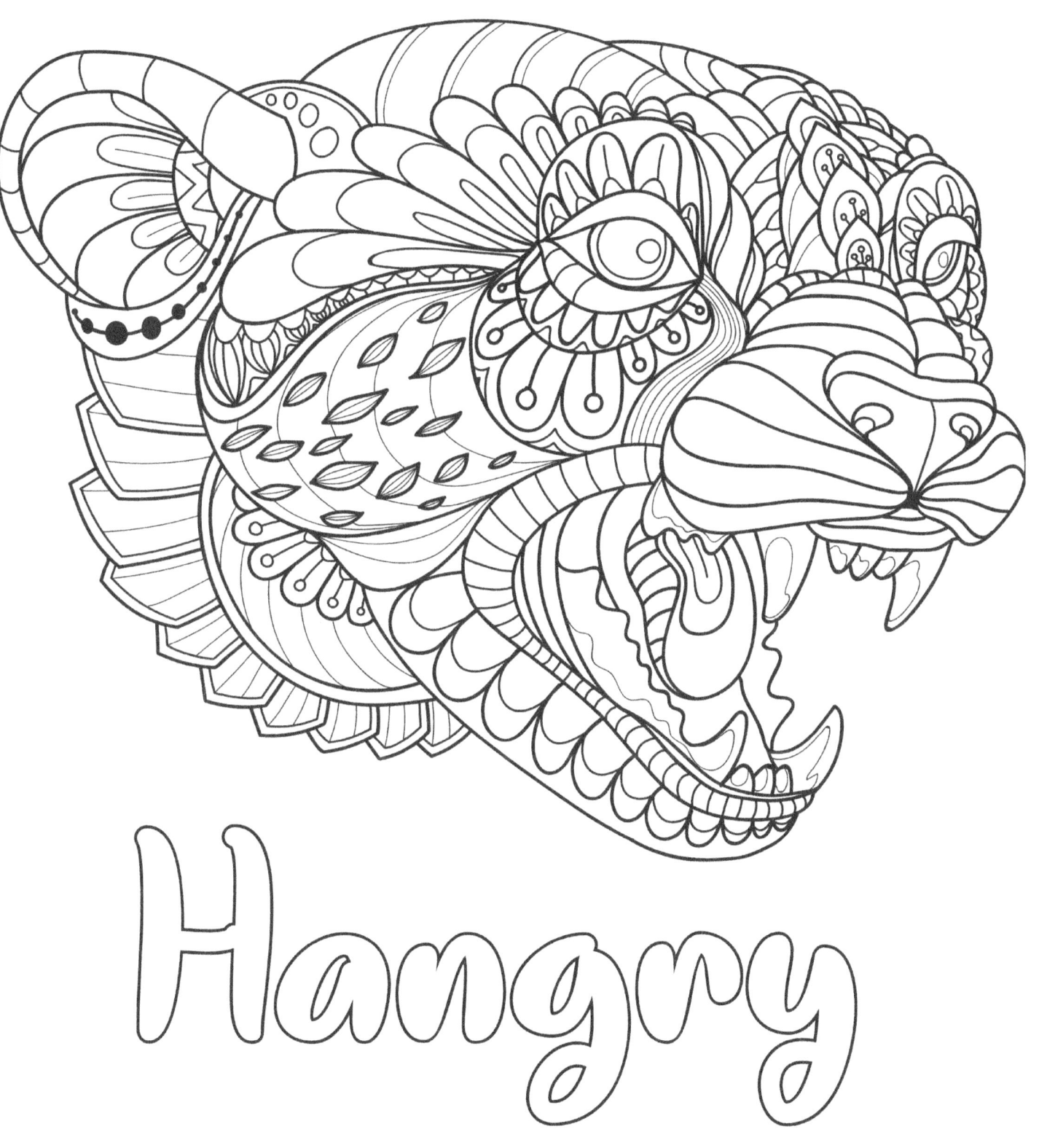

Hangry

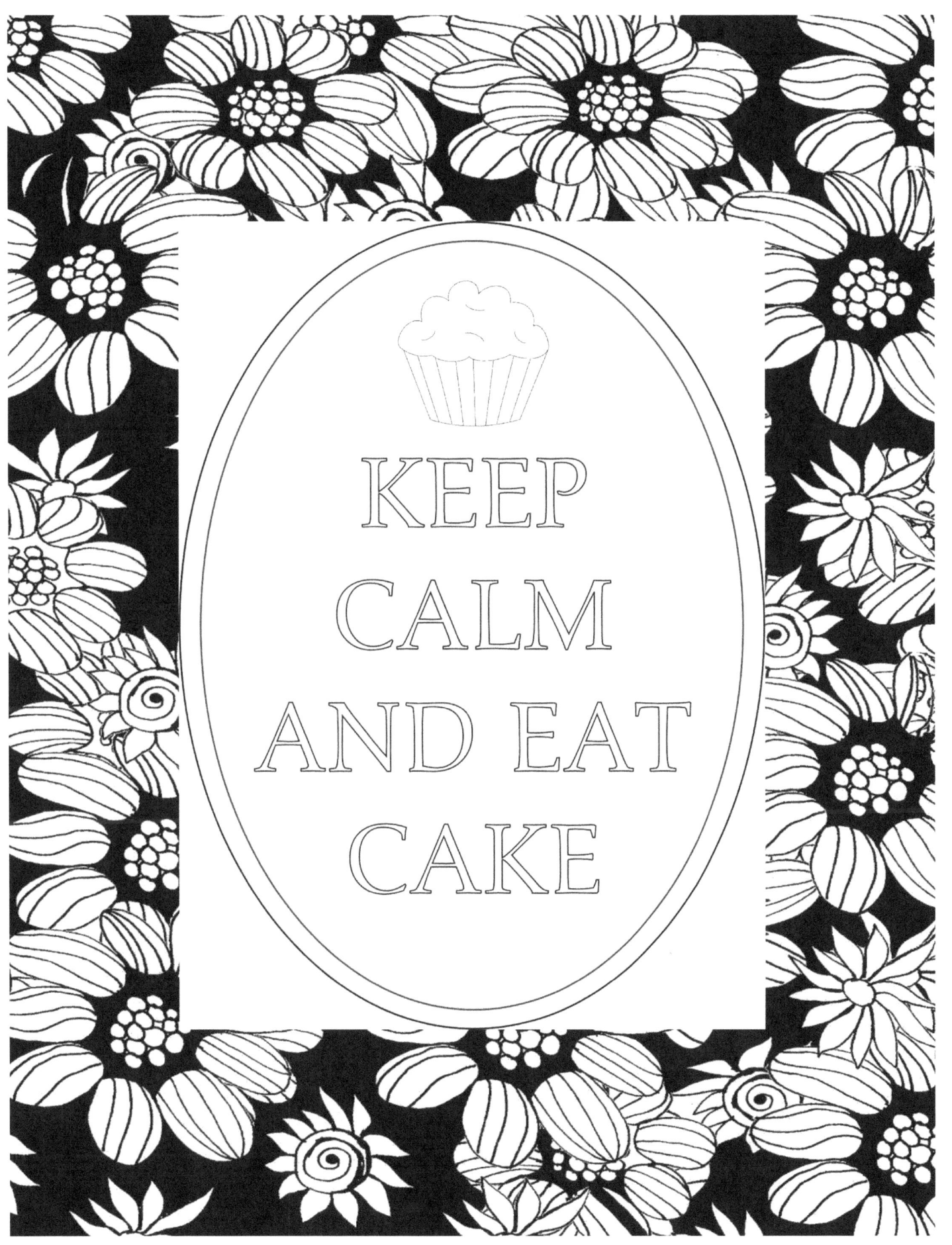

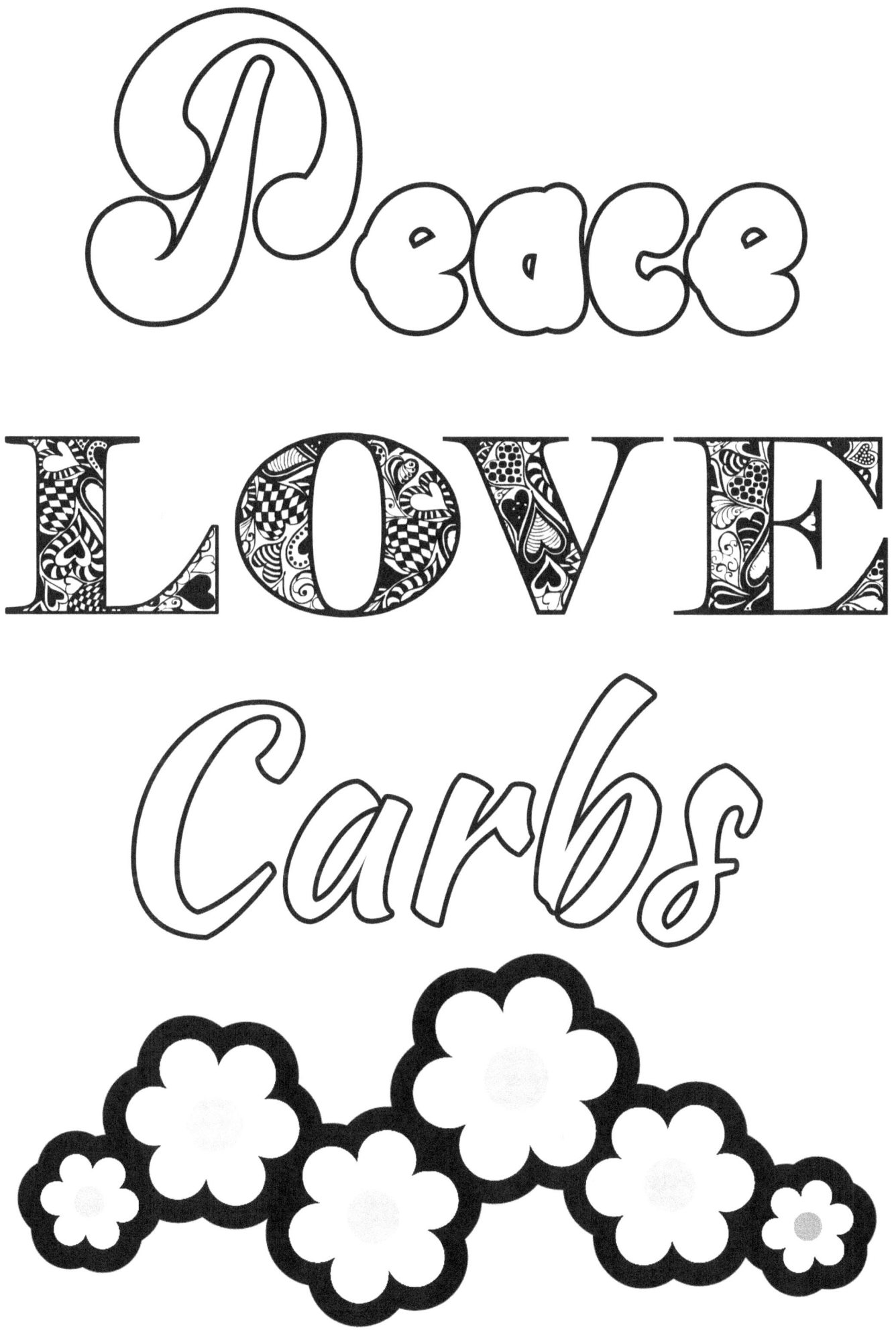

Body By

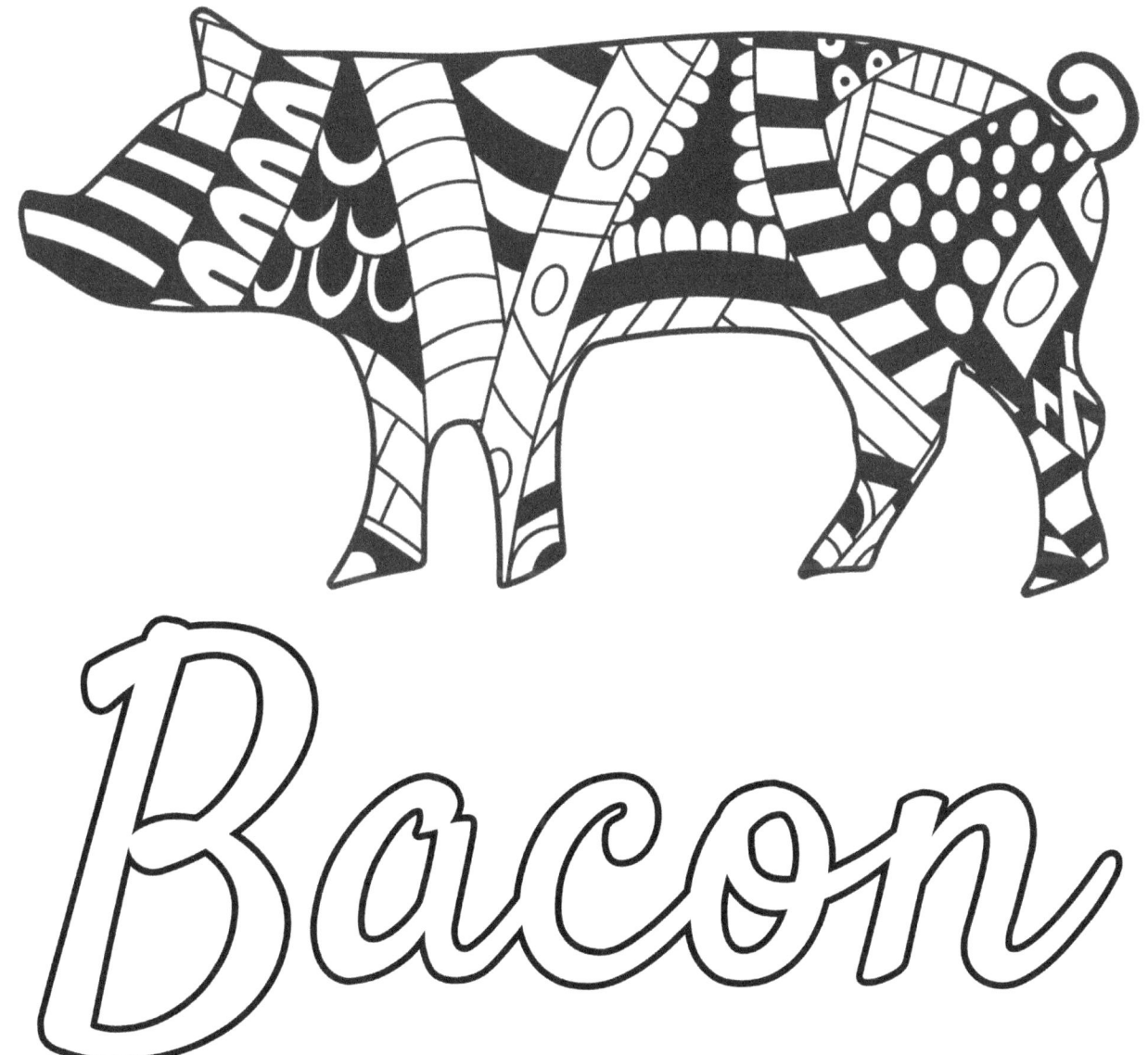

Bacon

Nobody Wants to Hear about

YOUR DIET.

JUST EAT YOUR SALAD & BE SAD...

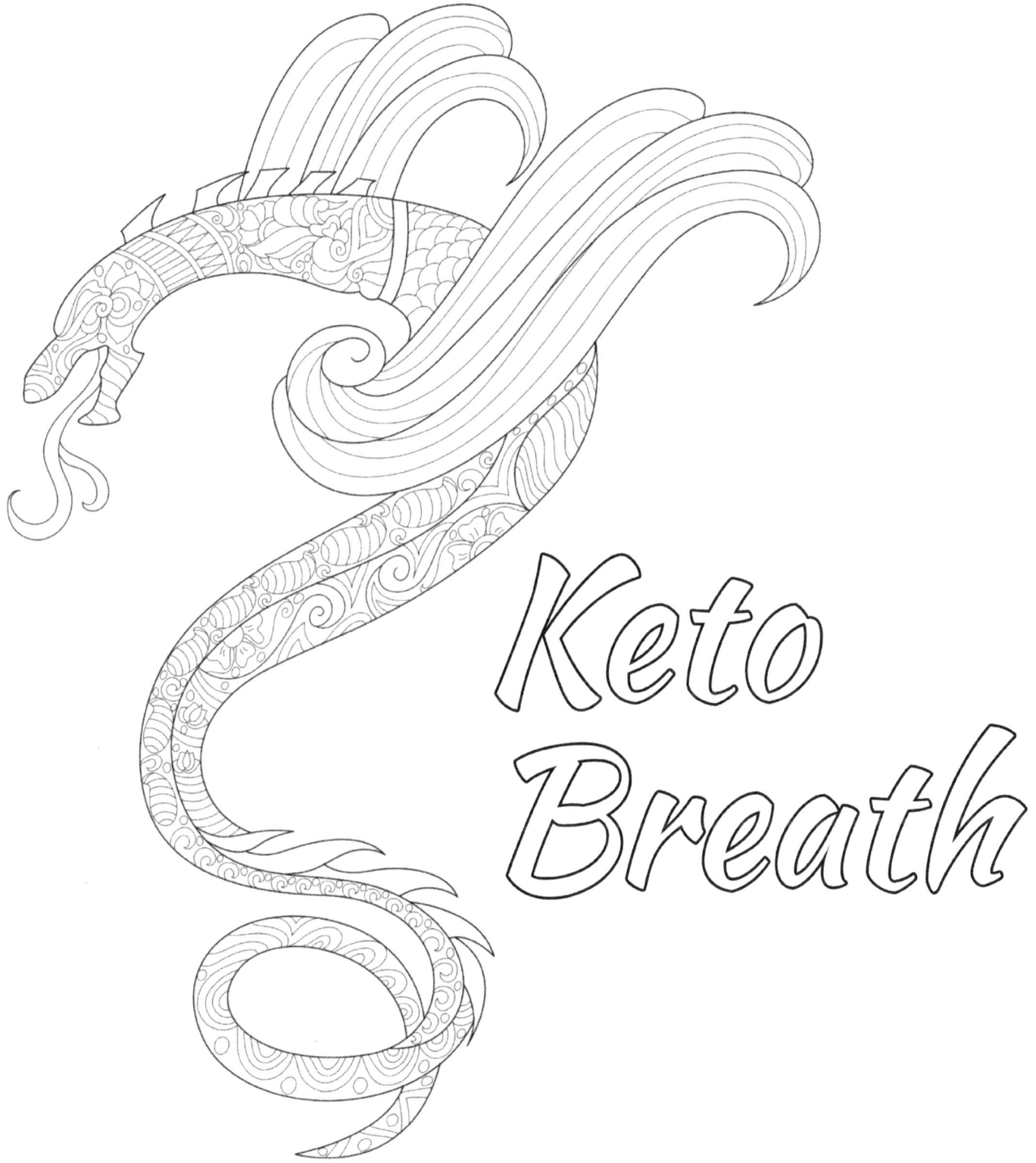

Keto
Breath

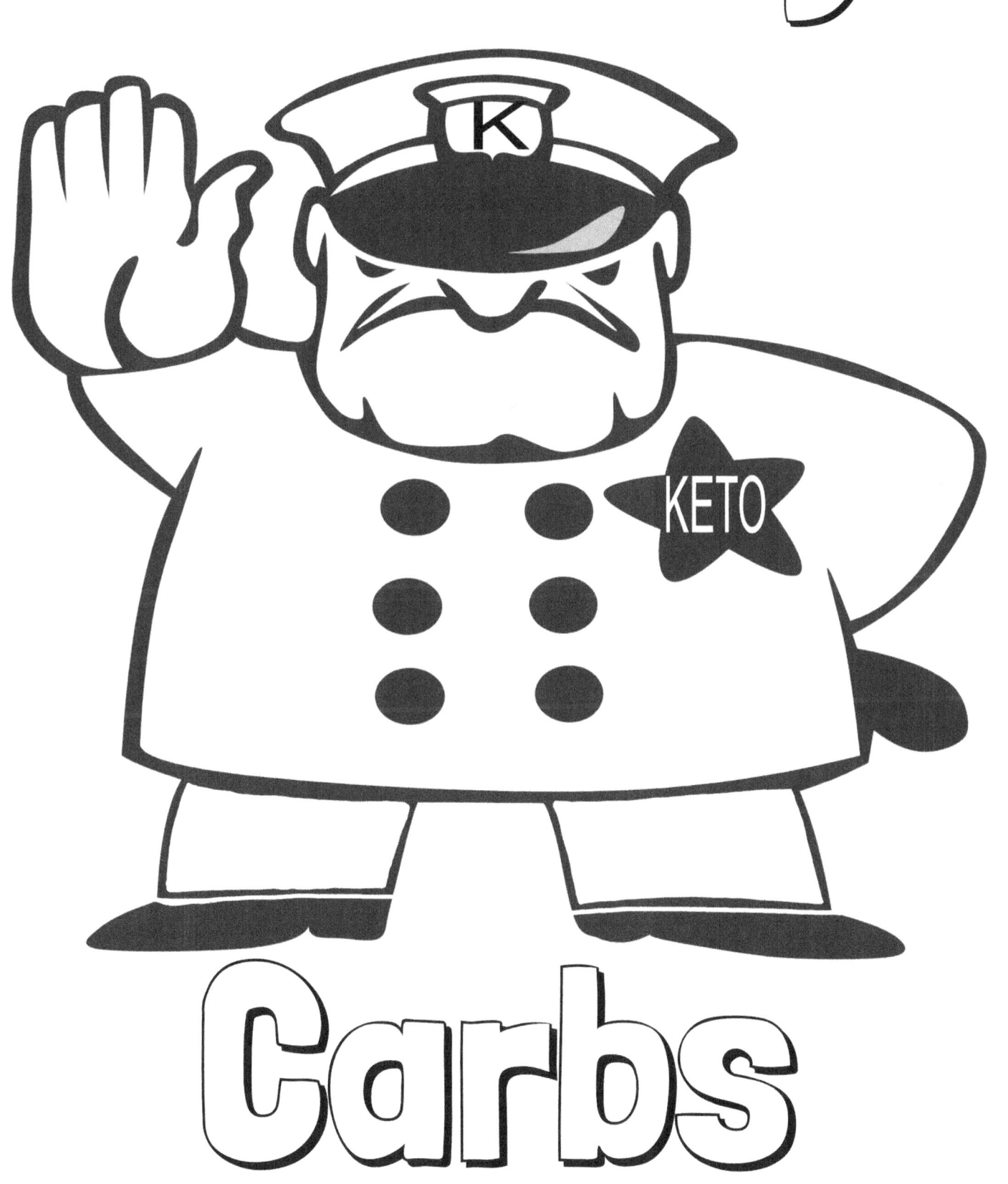

KETONES

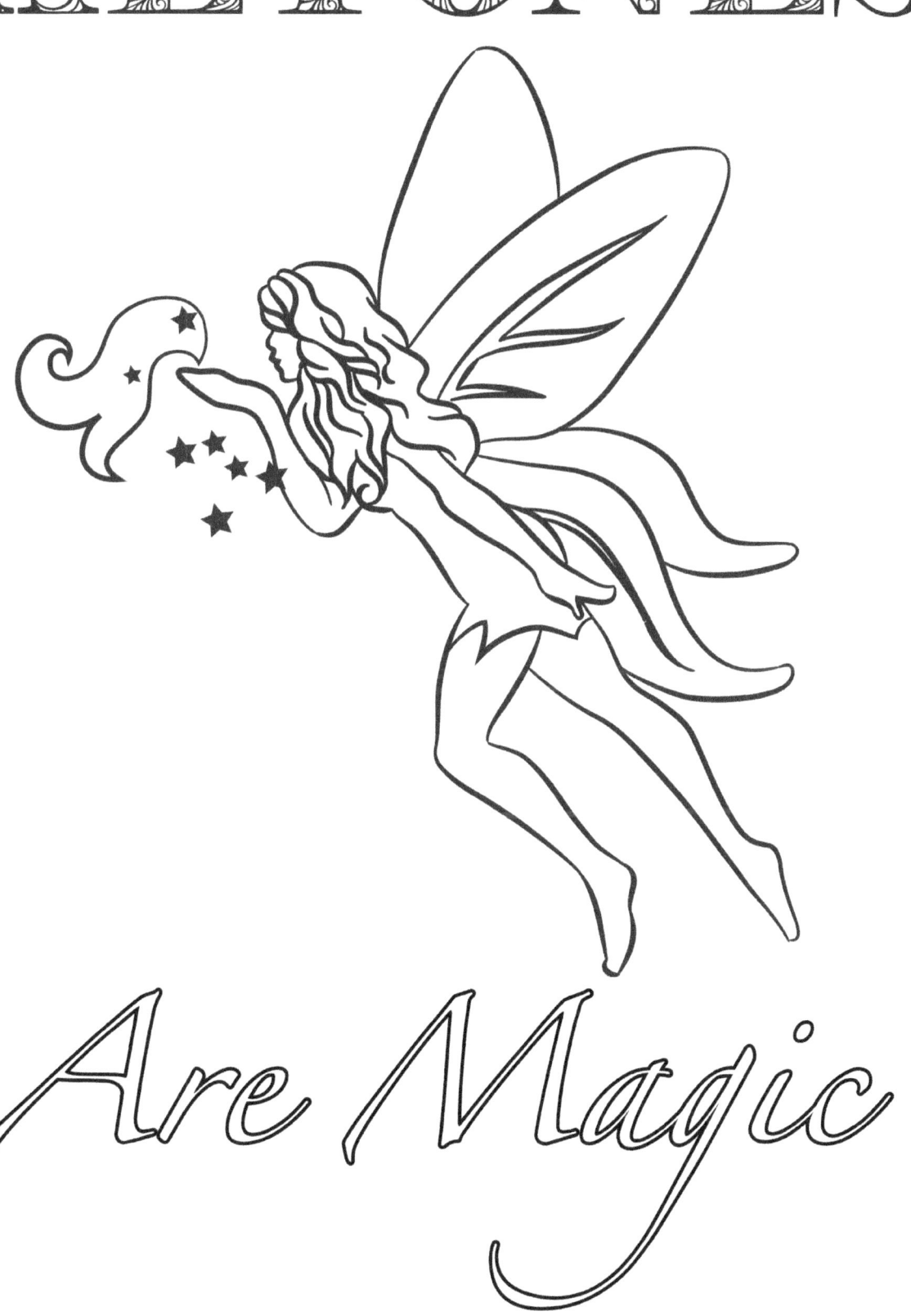

Are Magic

Other books from Cora Delmonico:

Volleyball Coloring Book & More
Softball Coloring Book
Another Mandala Coloring Book
This Weather can suck it!

Thank you for your purchase.

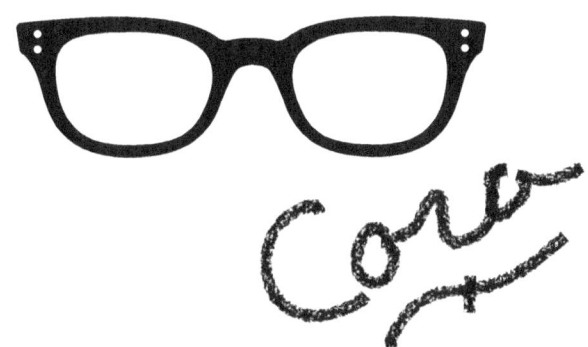